the BariatricBible

Your Essential Companion to Weight Loss Surgery

Carol Bowen Ball

THE EXPERIMENT

NEW YORK

The Experiment, LLC
220 East 23rd Street, Suite 600
New York, NY 10010-4658
theexperimentpublishing.com

This book contains the opinions and ideas of its author. It is intended to provide helpful and
informative material on the subjects addressed in the book. It is sold with the understanding that
the author and publisher are not engaged in rendering medical, health, or any other kind of
personal professional services in the book. The author and publisher specifically disclaim all
responsibility for any liability, loss, or risk—personal or otherwise—that is incurred as a
consequence, directly or indirectly, of the use and application of any of the contents of this book.

THE EXPERIMENT and its colophon are registered trademarks of The Experiment, LLC.
Many of the designations used by manufacturers and sellers to distinguish their products are
claimed as trademarks. Where those designations appear in this book and The Experiment was
aware of a trademark claim, the designations have been capitalized.

The Experiment's books are available at special discounts when purchased in bulk for premiums
and sales promotions as well as for fund-raising or educational use. For details, contact us at
info@theexperimentpublishing.com.

Library of Congress Cataloging-in-Publication Data available upon request

ISBN 978-1-61519-651-7
Ebook ISBN 978-1-61519-652-4

Cover design by Beth Bugler
Text design by Daniele Roa
Additional text design by Jack Dunnington
Food styling by Kathy Kordalis
Author photograph by Kate Griffin Photography

Manufactured in China

First printing April 2020
10 9 8 7 6 5 4 3 2 1

Contents

Foreword
by Neil Floch, MD, FACS

The journey of weight loss surgery must include the ownership of the quintessential guide for patients to follow. *The Bariatric Bible* is a remarkable creation that should be studied by every patient seeking to understand the procedures and the instructions involved before, during, and after bariatric surgery. It provides a pathway for the bariatric patient to live a life where eating food can be a healthy and pleasurable experience. *The Bariatric Bible* is a masterpiece of the most significant information, combining incredible photography that is almost as delicious to look at as the recipes are to eat. The book is highly successful in the United Kingdom and has now crossed the Atlantic to the shores of the US to nourish the American bariatric community.

As a bariatric surgeon who works in both private practice and academia, I can attest to the importance of this precious book, which serves as a guide to use throughout the bariatric surgery process. It explains bariatric information in terms that patients can visualize and understand. It is a bible for life.

Carol Bowen Ball has developed a passion for the bariatric patient, which led her to create the essential diet that is healthy and a joy to experience, enabling the bariatric patient to help achieve long-term weight loss. Her website, bariatriccookery.com, and her newsletter both serve as a guide to seventeen thousand bariatric patients a month. She has lucid insight into the needs of the bariatric patient, which is evident from the outstanding quality of her healthy and delicious recipes.

Carol is a self-taught master who has acquired vast knowledge of food preparation and bariatric nutrition. After undergoing gastric bypass surgery and maintaining a 100-pound weight loss, she has gained the wisdom to succeed—and now, she provides that knowledge to her readers for their success.

In this masterful scripture of more than two hundred written pages, Carol provides invaluable advice, inviting illustrations, beautiful photography, and outstanding recipes for her enticingly delicious food.

The first hundred pages of this bible include an extensive explanation of the bariatric surgery journey, with basic explanations of the procedures, the surgical preparation, and the recovery experience. Highlights of the first section include the basics of the bariatric diet and getting organized in the kitchen, and facts about warning foods, portion control, coping mechanisms, regain and plateaus, eating and travel, and coping with holidays.

Carol also includes details that only a bariatric surgery patient could understand and appreciate. Hers is a unique, accurate, and invaluable perspective that sets *The Bariatric Bible* apart from other books.

The second section of *The Bariatric Bible* is a treasure chest of two hundred pages, filled with recipes that are a testimony to healthy bariatric eating. The cookbook categorizes recipes into three stages: Liquids, Soft Food, and, as Carol delightfully puts it, "Food for Life," which are the components of the classic post-bariatric surgery diet. All the recipes are color-coded for simplicity and organized into breakfast, lunch, and dinner. Extending one step further, there are categories of dressings, desserts, vegetables, snacks, baking, drinks, and food for the holidays.

The recipes are easy to follow and contain post-surgery portions as well as regular portions, with calculations of calories, and carbohydrates, fats, and, most importantly, protein content. The information will help patients create menus that include the recipes they can easily follow, enjoy, and use to achieve weight loss success. It may tempt readers to substitute shakes and protein bars, and indulge instead in high-protein treats, such as Cheesy Jello Pots—with only 37 calories and 6.6 grams of protein. Reviewing the nutritional content is a learning experience that will surprise readers into knowing that delicious food can also be healthy.

It is an honor to present this consummate bible as a pathway to a healthy life after bariatric surgery. I commend Carol for her outstanding artistry and illuminating achievement in presenting an extraordinary wealth of information in this definitive book for the bariatric patient, *The Bariatric Bible*.

NEIL FLOCH, MD, FACS, is director of bariatric surgery at Norwalk Hospital and Danbury Hospital, Nuvance Health, Connecticut, and associate clinical professor of surgery at the Robert Larner College of Medicine at the University of Vermont.

Preface

Bariatric or weight loss surgery (WLS) is a lifesaver, new-life-giver, and game-changer, as thousands of patients around the world will attest. I feel fortunate to have been one of them and to have met so many others who have also experienced the journey.

My journey began many years ago when I simply ran out of ideas for how to deal with my weight. Years of constant yo-yo dieting didn't help, but I also believed my body was in conflict with my mind about shedding its excess weight. Believe me, I tried so many times to persuade it to think otherwise. The final solution, I hoped, would be bariatric surgery. I was seduced by the opportunity for my body (and perhaps my mind) to have a reset, and have one final go at getting things right.

I had a gastric bypass and lost and then maintained an almost 100-pound reduction in my weight. But (and there always is a "but" isn't there?), it hasn't been easy. I work at it every day and will undoubtedly continue to do so for the rest of my life. I am proud of my weight loss but even prouder of my maintenance.

While my previous journeys into weight loss had been tricky, this was definitely new terrain for me to negotiate. I had to deal not only with the surgery itself but also a new challenging eating regimen in order to stay fit and well. Add to that the complexities of medications, an exercise regimen, and coping with a whole change of life scenario, and it has been a huge, sharp learning curve. Plus, as a food writer, I needed to get to grips with cooking and selecting food in a different way.

Luckily, along the road, I had the help of an amazing bariatric team, supportive family and friends, as well as new WLS friends and helpful professional contacts in the bariatric surgery field. This, I believe, along with my commitment, resolve, and compliance, has been the key to success.

I have learned a great deal since my surgery. The website I set up to help others—bariatriccookery. com—has given me additional professional contacts, too. Through their guest posts, they have unselfishly given their time and energy to helping not only me but also many others on this road to recovery from obesity. Their features on subjects that are complex and specialized (which they have kindly allowed me to share with you) are so valuable when the WLS community is so poorly underserved. I hope my recipes and food advice prove just as useful.

The *Bariatric Bible* is an attempt to crystallize and condense all of this information—and ambitiously be the first and last word on negotiating a bariatric lifestyle. A tall order, but I hope we have covered the salient facts and also provided some inspiration on how to eat and enjoy your food after surgery.

I am constantly asked what my tips for success are, and they are many and varied, but in a nutshell I would say make food your friend not your enemy. It's just food! I know life gets in the way but make realistic plans, keep your motivation alive, don't become phobic about certain food groups (carbs and fats aren't all bad), try to trash your triggers and unhealthy temptations, create a great support system, move as much as you can, be adventurous with food choices, and finally, take care of yourself (which may mean practicing a bit more self-care and love).

I'm with you on this.

Carol Bowen Ball

Introduction

All across the world, in the media, on the agenda of governments, in research papers and journals, in hospitals and boardrooms, the rising level of obesity is being discussed and debated. This rising tide is of huge concern not only because of a nation's health but also because it has huge impact on the planning of services, the effectiveness of a workforce, and the costs implicated with this. The impact on overstretched health services has been laid bare and is most worrying—not least because it now has been identified within the young population, too.

WHAT IS OBESITY?
At the very simplest level, obesity is defined as a Body Mass Index (BMI) of over 30. The BMI is a common measure of obesity that provides a comparison of an individual's weight in relation to their height and is strongly associated with body fat percentage.

WHAT CAUSES OBESITY?
Those taking a simplistic view often say it's just a matter of individuals eating too much—or an energy imbalance—the disparity between energy taken in as food, and energy expended out. The more enlightened know that many other factors also come into play—those relating to genetic, sociological, technological, and individual motivators.

It is said that genes are responsible for 70 percent of a person's weight gain. These genes control factors as diverse as appetite, satiety, and metabolism, with all the complexities and vagaries they involve. Factor in differences of willpower, lifestyle choice, and food availability, for example, and you have the makings of a very complex scenario that can't be explained in a simple in/out equation. The behavior patterns resulting from all these components ensure that is so.

Anyone who has struggled with excess pounds will recognize that with weight management there isn't a "one size fits all" solution. Many have tried to find the answer as the countless number of "miracle" diets that are touted testify. What we do know is that they have limited success and often fail. Only a mere 5 percent of dieters lose their excess weight and keep it off long term. The residual 95 percent tend to yo-yo between one diet and another and often start the next one heavier than the previous one.

THE IMPLICATIONS OF OBESITY
In a nutshell, obesity is disabling—from minor to severe. At its simplest, it can shorten a person's lifespan by several years. The cost to an individual is therefore very significant, but it's also costly to a nation. There are economic costs through loss of work, incapacity benefits, and increasing health-care needs of those who are too ill to work.

WHAT CAN SOLVE IT?
There are as many suggested solutions as there are diets. For some, the final option is bariatric or weight loss surgery. This is usually considered when all the usual, more conservative methods have been tried without success. Surgery is often mentioned as the "last solution."

Bariatric surgery is known to be the most effective and long-lasting treatment for morbid obesity (those with a BMI over 40) and its many related conditions. There is also mounting evidence to demonstrate that it also may be among the most effective treatments for other metabolic diseases, including obstructive sleep apnea, Type 2 diabetes, hypertension, nonalcoholic fatty liver disease, and high cholesterol. It's also considered cost effective, since the cost of most operations can be "paid for" in terms of reduced medications and state benefits and increased work input when there is a return to work.

But surgery for the morbidly obese goes way beyond weight loss, for not only are comorbidities and life-limiting diseases improved, but others, like asthma, fertility, and mental health–related issues, can also be improved or resolved. More importantly, unlike diets, the effects are long-lasting.

Of course, surgery isn't a complete cure, and some will continue the battle against weight gain with sensible eating and lifestyle changes. Surgery is simply the tool that helps them to reinforce these dietary changes and makes them easier to accomplish. For most severely obese patients, it is all they need to lead a happy, healthier, and more fulfilling life.

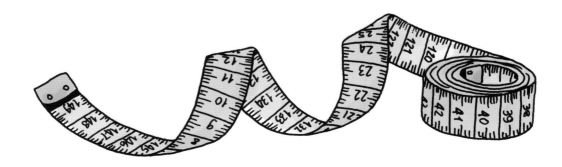

PART ONE

The Procedure

Bariatric Surgery

Bariatric surgery is only the start to the solution of obesity, for once you've had the surgery, then the real work begins. The surgery can be a "reset" but it's essentially a tool to help and assist with weight loss.

After the procedure and recuperation, there is still much work to be done on developing a new dietary regimen, employing coping mechanisms for compliance, and dealing with all the emotional issues that may still linger or arise through weight control. Old habits die hard.

In short, many aspects of a WLS patient's life will change, and the surgery is not a "magic wand" to deal with them all. Most surgeons quote that they do the mechanics but the patient then does the after-work and day-to-day care to ensure smooth running of the newly altered system.

Those who criticize the WLS patient for "taking the easy way out" or who consider this surgery a "cheat" are seriously deluded. WLS afterlife is hard work, relentless, and challenging. The surgery itself is just the beginning—what you do afterwards is the real key to success.

What Types Are Available?

Bariatric or Weight Loss Surgery (WLS) can be a gastric balloon, gastric band, gastric bypass, gastric sleeve, duodenal switch, or other revision surgery.

All the main operations are good and have impressive success rates. However, the people who get matched with the best operation for them,

who sort out their aftercare and make ongoing lifestyle and dietary changes, are the people who consistently have the best long-term results.

Here are the main procedures that you and your surgeon may consider:

GASTRIC BALLOON

The gastric balloon device is often associated with weight loss surgery but in fact is not truly a surgical procedure. The gastric balloon is a highly-effective form of non-surgical weight loss intervention. It is recommended for patients who are overweight, which is defined as having a Body Mass Index (BMI) of 27 or more, and who have struggled to lose weight through diet and exercise alone.

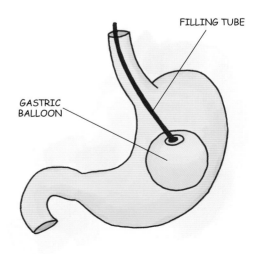

FILLING TUBE

GASTRIC
BALLOON

How It Works: The gastric balloon is a soft silicone sac that is placed in the stomach. It is inserted empty and then filled using sterile saline. Once in place, the balloon takes up volume in the stomach, so that the patient needs to eat much less before the stomach sends "feeling full" signals to the brain. The patient therefore stops eating sooner and consumes fewer calories. The balloon stays in place for six months, after which time it is deflated and removed.

The Benefits: Patients can expect to lose up to 42 pounds (19 kg) in the first six months. It is a good option for patients who are looking to kick-start their diet and healthy-eating regimen that they will then carry on themselves.

The gastric balloon is also sometimes used for morbidly obese patients who need to lose weight before having a bypass or sleeve procedure, which is invasive surgery. As the balloon is not a surgical procedure, recovery is much faster and the procedure is deemed much safer, requiring no anesthetic.

The procedure is normally carried out under light sedation. It is a relatively straightforward outpatient surgery and normally requires no overnight stay.

The Diet: In order to be successful with the gastric balloon, patients need to commit to change their dietary habits for life. The balloon is a useful tool to start the process. The bariatric team will advise on the diet to follow and good food choices to make.

GASTRIC BAND

The gastric band, also know as the "lapband," is a surgical solution recommended for patients who are overweight or obese with a BMI over 35 (or 30 if there are other comorbidites, such as diabetes, or obesity-related concerns).

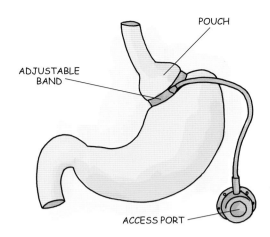

POUCH

ADJUSTABLE BAND

ACCESS PORT

How It Works: The gastric band works to restrict the amount a person can eat by reducing their appetite and reducing the stomach's capacity. The band device is placed around the top of the stomach to divide it into a characteristic hour-glass shape. The top part of the stomach feels full faster. Food then passes into the lower section of the stomach and is then digested as normal. The patient feels fuller sooner, and for longer, and therefore loses weight simply by eating less.

The Benefits: The key benefit of the gastric band over other forms of surgery is that it is adjustable and even reversible. Adjustability means that the patient's weight loss can be controlled. In the early months, the band will be tightened a number of times after surgery to provide greater restriction on the stomach (see page 20). Once the weight loss target has been reached, the band will usually be loosened slightly to provide optimal restriction (often called the "sweet spot") so that weight loss can be maintained for the long term.

Gastric band surgery is normally carried out under general anesthetic as a laparoscopic, or "keyhole," procedure. Patients should expect to spend a night in the hospital before leaving to recover at home.

The Diet: A staged gastric band diet will be advised by the bariatric team. First, before surgery, patients are usually required to follow a pre-op regimen to reduce the size of their liver to make surgery as safe and straightforward as possible.

After surgery, patients initially follow a liquid diet, gradually progressing through a puréed diet, and then eventually to a normal diet.

GASTRIC SLEEVE

The gastric sleeve, also known as "sleevectomy" and "vertical sleeve gastrectomy" is now perhaps one of the most popular WLS procedures in the world, along with the gastric bypass. It is a highly effective form of surgery that is recommended for patients with a BMI of 35 or more.

How It Works: The gastric sleeve procedure involves removing part of the stomach to create a smaller, slimmer stomach pouch, which has a characteristic "sleeve shape." After surgery, a smaller stomach means that there is a smaller capacity for food, so patients feel full sooner and for longer. In addition, the part of the stomach that is removed is associated with the production of the hunger hormone ghrelin, so this further represses the patient's appetite.

The Benefits: The key benefit of the gastric sleeve is that it is a less invasive form of surgery compared to the gastric bypass, yet offers more aggressive weight loss results than the gastric band for those patients that fall into the severely obese or morbidly obese categories.

Gastric sleeve surgery is normally carried out under general anesthetic as a laparoscopic, or "keyhole," procedure, although in certain cases an "open procedure" may be undertaken. Patients should expect to spend two to three nights in the hospital, before leaving to recover at home.

The gastric sleeve may also be converted to a

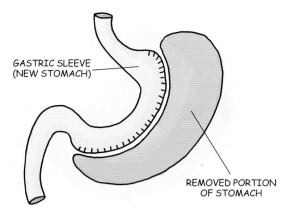

GASTRIC SLEEVE (NEW STOMACH)

REMOVED PORTION OF STOMACH

gastric bypass later. For some patients it is performed as "step 1," enabling them to lose weight and be healthier before the full gastric bypass is completed.

The good news is that after weight loss, obesity-related conditions, such as Type 2 diabetes, high blood pressure or sleep apnea, can be expected to improve considerably and even go into remission.

The Diet: A staged gastric sleeve diet will be advised by the bariatric team. Before surgery, patients are usually required to follow a pre-op diet to reduce the size of the liver to make surgery as safe and straightforward as possible. After surgery, patients initially follow a liquid diet, gradually progressing through a puréed diet, to a soft food diet, and finally a normal diet. Throughout these stages, it is vital to follow medical advice. Patients will be consuming fewer calories, so it is essential that good food choices for optimum nutrition are made.

In addition, gastric sleeve patients will be required to take supplements, vitamins, and minerals for the rest of their life. Blood tests on a regular basis are also recommended so that any deficiencies are spotted early and can be rectified.

GASTRIC BYPASS

The gastric bypass is the most invasive of all the popular weight loss surgery procedures but it offers the greatest potential weight loss. It is suited to those with a significant amount of weight to lose and offers excellent clinically-proven results.

It is recommended for patients who are overweight or obese with a BMI over 40, which is defined as "morbidly obese." At this weight, the patient often has obesity-related conditions, such as Type 2 diabetes, high blood pressure, or sleep apnea. This makes losing weight a high priority to improve the patient's health and quality of life.

How It Works: The gastric bypass procedure involves creating a new stomach pouch the size of a golf ball or egg, which limits the amount a patient can eat. Then, a section of small intestine is attached to the stomach pouch, allowing food to bypass most of the small intestine so that the body's absorption of calories and nutrients is significantly reduced.

The procedure works on two levels. Due to the small stomach capacity, the patient will be far less hungry and eat much smaller portions, as they will feel satisfied very quickly when eating. In addition, due to the bypass, the food that they do eat will be absorbed less readily by the body. Therefore, gastric bypass patients achieve high levels of weight loss.

The Diet: A staged gastric bypass diet will be advised by the bariatric team. Before having surgery, patients are usually required to follow a pre-op diet to reduce the size of their liver to make surgery as safe and straightforward as possible. After surgery, patients initially follow a liquid diet, gradually progressing through a puréed diet, to a soft food diet, and finally a normal diet. Throughout these stages, it is vital to follow medical advice. Patients will be consuming and absorbing fewer calories, so it is essential that good food choices for optimum nutrition are made. A healthier, balanced diet is essential after gastric bypass surgery.

In addition, gastric bypass patients will be required to take supplements, vitamins, and minerals for the rest of their life. Blood tests on a regular basis are also recommended so that any deficiencies are spotted early and can be rectified.

MINI GASTRIC BYPASS

The mini gastric bypass procedure has gained popularity in recent years. It is a procedure that is restrictive and malabsorptive. This means the procedure reduces the size of the stomach, restricting the amount you can eat and reducing absorption of food by bypassing up to six feet of intestine. It has been developed to reduce operating time, simplify the procedure, and reduce complications. At present, it is not covered by all insurance carriers and so may not be an option for some patients. It also has the additional risk of severe acid reflux. Because the pouch is small, and the remainder of the stomach is still connected to the intestines, it is possible for gastric juices to travel down the intestines and into the new pouch. Recovery is very similar to traditional gastric bypass surgery.

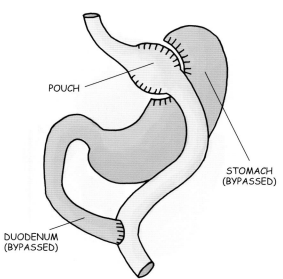

POUCH

STOMACH (BYPASSED)

DUODENUM (BYPASSED)

DUODENAL SWITCH

The duodenal switch (DS) procedure, also known as biliopancreatic diversion with duodenal switch (BPD-DS) or gastric reduction duodenal switch (GRDS), is a weight loss surgery procedure that has both restrictive and malabsorptive aspects.

It is a specialized procedure and requires huge lifestyle changes.

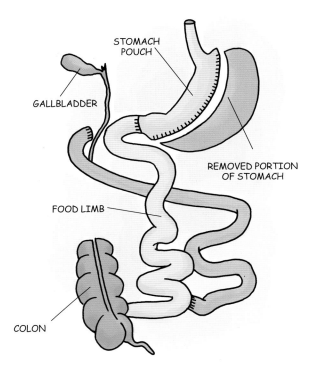

The Route to Bariatric Surgery

The route to bariatric surgery generally takes two forms: a self-funded pathway (paid for by the patient or their private insurance provider, which can take place at home or abroad), or a state-funded public type.

IS MORBID OBESITY OR OBESITY COVERED BY YOUR INDIVIDUAL POLICY?

The best way to check this is to contact your insurance provider—often this information can be found on the back of your insurance card. If it is a covered benefit, then check that the procedure and surgery type you are considering is also provided—sometimes not all are. At this stage, it is undoubtedly useful to ask what percentage of the total bill you will be responsible for, and if you will need to pay a deductible, and if there are any specific criteria you need to meet for consideration.

SOME COMMON REQUIREMENTS FOR WLS INSURANCE COVERAGE

Insurance providers may have different requirements for their coverage of WLS. Criteria can be mandated by your employer or a medical policy, or be plan-specific.

Common requirements are as follows:
- You are over age eighteen (but some plans do allow for surgery under the age of eighteen).
- You have a BMI over 40; or over 35 with other risk factors such as diabetes or high blood pressure.
- You have documented weight loss efforts over a period of time.
- You have undergone psychological testing.
- You have attended a weight loss program mandated by the insurance company.
- You quit smoking prior to surgery.
- You have no evidence of substance abuse.
- You receive a diagnosis of morbid obesity for a specific period of time prior to surgery.

WHO FOOTS THE BILL FOR THIS?

Many insurance companies, both public and private now offer coverage for bariatric surgery. It does, however, vary widely by state and insurance provider. The first step to consider is contacting your insurance company to find out if the procedure you would like is covered, and what caveats, if any, may exist. Many have strict requirements (some less stringent) and some will foot the entire bill (while others, only part or a percentage of it).

MEDICARE AND WLS

Medicare, the US government health plan, typically requires candidates to take part in a six-month medically-supervised weight loss program through their bariatric surgeon or their primary care physician before they will cover the cost of WLS. Find out the specific requirements regarding your dietary history by contacting your local Medicare provider. Currently, WLS is an option for those with a body mass index (BMI) of 35, with at least one health problem relating to their obesity such as diabetes or heart disease. Medicare does mandate that the WLS takes place at a specifically certified location. However, Medicare does not require pre-certification or pre-authorization of medical necessity from a doctor before they agree to pay for WLS—unlike that required by many private insurers.

In the case of Medicare, a surgeon will submit the claim after the patient has met all the Medicare requirements for WLS. Some surgeons may ask Medicare patients to sign a contract stating they will pay for any costs that Medicare does not cover after the claim is processed.

MEDICAID AND WLS

Medicaid is the federal government's health care plan for certain low-income families and individuals. Whether Medicaid offers and covers WLS varies on a state-by-state basis and can be a bit of a zip-code lottery. Some states are very progressive and proactive and some not so much.

PRIVATE INSURANCE COMPANIES AND WLS

Many US private insurance companies will cover WLS if your primary care doctor informs them that the surgery is medically necessary. That said, the patient must back this up with good medical and other documentation to validate the case.

In general, most private insurance companies require a letter of medical necessity from your WLS surgeon and your primary care physician in order to be considered. This letter should include the following information:

- your height, weight, weight history, and BMI
- a detailed description of your obesity-related health conditions, including records of treatment (such conditions might include diabetes, heart disease, high blood pressure, sleep apnea, and gastroesophageal reflux)
- a list of your current medications
- a detailed description and analysis of how obesity affects your everyday activities, health, and life
- a detailed history of your past dieting efforts to date; a number of insurers now require detailed documentation of attendance and participation of the candidate in a physician-supervised plan—most require submissions of at least six months' worth of notes detailing this from a supervising doctor
- a history of exercise programs and lifestyle change efforts, along with gym membership documentation as proof of engagement, prior to consideration of surgery.

HOW CAN YOU IMPROVE YOUR CHANCES OF INSURANCE COVERAGE

It may seem like your chances are in the lap of the gods, but there is much that you can do to improve your chances of getting insurance coverage. Collect (and keep in a safe place) all letters and documentation from all the health care professionals who have treated you for your health conditions related to obesity. These may be the springboard

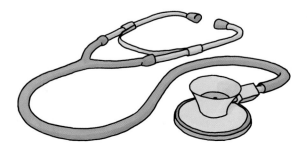

you need to start the process. Many insurers also require a nutritional and psychological evaluation. Talk to your surgeon about referrals during early visits, so that you are not left waiting for them.

It cannot be underestimated how important it is to get your bariatric physician and surgeon on board during this time. Many know the ins and outs of multiple insurance carriers—with them in tandem or alongside you, the process can be easier and pitfalls can be reduced or erased.

Some bariatric physicians also offer special payment plans—talk to them about this in the early stages, so that you can budget carefully.

Not all candidates are successful, and coverage is occasionally denied. But you can appeal, and you should immediately initiate your appeal. Each insurance company has an appeal process—check this ahead of time, so you're not set back if you face this disappointment.

A Few More Tips

Choosing a surgeon for your WLS can be one of the biggest decisions you make on the journey. You may not have much choice if you're in an HMO or your insurance limits your options. If you're self-pay, or in some PPOs, or other healthcare plans, you may have tons of choices. How can you get the surgeon that will you give you the tools you need to lose weight successfully?

The following are some of the basic tips for choosing a surgeon:

- Choose one with plenty of experience.
- Read reviews.
- Ask for recommendations from your primary care doctor and any friends or family members who are WLS patients.
- Find out about follow-up care and dietary support.
- Use your gut instinct. It's often good at telling which surgeon is right for you.

DO YOU UNDERSTAND EVERYTHING?

Communication is a big part of WLS success. You need to understand what is happening to you and what your surgeon and nutritionist ask you to do. When choosing a surgeon, ask all of your questions about the procedure and the aftercare.

Don't blame yourself if you don't understand your surgeon's answers. It's your surgeon's job to explain everything in terms you can understand. If you can't understand, and can't get the surgeon to explain, it may be time for you to move on. This is too important a decision to risk going with someone who cannot communicate.

THIS IS AS GOOD AS IT GETS

It's only natural to think things will get better, but don't count on it when you're choosing a surgeon. If surgeons don't have time to meet with you and explain everything now, they won't have time later. If you can't get an appointment with the nutritionist now, it's not going to be any easier later.

In short, surgeons are putting their best foot forward when they're trying to get you to commit to surgery with them. If they're not satisfying you now, they're not going to meet your expectations later. Find a surgeon who starts off by going beyond your expectations—plenty of outstanding surgeons are out there!

Going Abroad

In recent times we have seen an increase in "health tourism." It's possible for people to travel abroad or across borders to have surgery. This is an attractive option for many patients, particularly because the initial costs can appear to be cheaper. There are a lot of experienced surgeons throughout the world—some have even pioneered this kind of surgery. But I would advise you to travel for surgery only if you are a resident in the country where that surgeon works, so they could get to you quickly if problems were to develop.

Safety is the reason for this precaution. Safety doesn't just mean a safe operation; it means safe follow-up, and access to help in emergencies. The ability to afford commuting on a regular basis to the country where you had your operation is not widespread, I'm afraid. Many patients see surgery as a one-stop cure; they have the operation and trust everything will be all right. It's a sad fact that many commercial groups promote this false impression, and ultimately, patients pay the price. Let me be clear—if you do not have follow-up appointments, problems can and will occur. The money you saved by having the surgery abroad may be quickly swallowed up by the costs of "repair" when you're back on home soil. Finally, the healthcare systems abroad are not the same as the ones in the US. There are different credentialing schemes for surgeons and hospitals. If problems occur, could you navigate your way through the complaint system of a foreign hospital in a foreign language? Would you even know with whom to lodge a complaint? At least at home there are many hundreds of willing lawyers who specialize in medical negligence and who'd be more than delighted to help you!

So, I would not recommend surgery abroad— but if you are considering it, please ask your surgeon all the questions outlined earlier and get their responses in writing.

Mental Health Considerations

Many people having surgery for severe obesity also have mental health conditions, particularly depression and binge-eating disorder. Some suffer with mood-related disorders of varying degrees.

Bariatric teams recognize the importance of checking a candidate's mental health prior to surgery, since it is important that they be able to manage post-surgery changes that may be very challenging.

The good news is that studies have shown that weight loss is not hindered after surgery by those who display mental health problems. But the caveat is that the team and MDs do need to be aware of these mental health conditions and refer the patient for treatment if necessary.

It is therefore unsurprising that some kind of mental health screening takes place by most providers prior to surgery. This is typically done by a mental health professional who then advises if it is wise to move ahead and the course to take with subsequent evaluation on timings.

While this evaluation may take time, it is worthwhile, and it is important to note that a mental health diagnosis does not automatically disqualify someone from having WLS. It is important to be open about this.

A person with moderate depression would be managed quite differently from someone having suicidal thoughts, for example. The suicidal patient is unlikely to be a good candidate for surgery; the depressed patient may well have the procedure and receive depression therapy—both before and after, in the best case scenario.

In all cases, patients are recommended to talk through their symptoms and concerns relating to mental health when accessing surgery. Mental health conditions should, in an ideal world, be considered another potential comorbidity of severe obesity, just like diabetes and high blood pressure.

Risks of Bariatric Surgery

For some, surgery can seem like an intimidating option. Making the decision to "go under the knife" can be nerve-racking and does take some consideration. But, with all of the benefits patients can gain from undergoing WLS, the results of surgery often outweigh the risks. If you're considering weight loss surgery or already have plans to undergo a bariatric procedure, here are some risks you should be aware of. Keep in mind that your risk level can only be determined by your healthcare providers.

Surgical complications: As with any surgery, there is always a risk of surgical complications— even with a minimally invasive procedure like WLS. These complications can include excessive bleeding, pulmonary embolism, gastrointestinal leak, and death. However, these complications only occur in about 1 percent of patients. Your risk level will also depend on your BMI (body mass index) and any severe medical conditions. Your surgeon will be able to assess your risk level based on your specific situation.

Post-surgery risks: Following surgery, complications can occur if patients don't follow their surgeon's instructions or if something went wrong with the procedure itself. Infection, nutritional deficiencies, failure to lose weight or maintain weight loss, too much weight loss, and other post-surgery complications are possible, although rare. Also, some surgeries have their own specific complications. For example, lap band patients may need to have their band adjusted a few times before they begin to lose weight at an appropriate rate.

Fertility and Pregnancy After WLS

WLS can affect fertility and your chances of getting pregnant as well as the pregnancy itself. If this affects you, you should know these seven facts.

- *You may get a boost in fertility:* WLS can produce a sudden positive change in your fertility. This newfound fertility can raise your chances of getting pregnant by accident if you haven't been using birth control, which can be a problem if you're in the initial eighteen-month post-op surgery period. You would be wise to check out your birth control options.

- *You should wait eighteen months before getting pregnant:* It's safe to get pregnant after WLS, after your weight stabilizes. After surgery, your body goes through stressful changes and significant nutritional upheaval, which can pose problems for a growing baby. To protect women and their babies from potential malnutrition, doctors recommend that women do not get pregnant until eighteen months after surgery. Ideally, a woman should have reached a stable weight and be able to provide her baby with enough nutrition.

- *You'll need to monitor your nutrient intake closely:* Nutritional deficiencies can be problematic because of low food intake and malabsorption issues, and nausea (a common pregnancy complication) can add to this. To make sure you and your baby are getting enough nutrients, it is important to see a nutritionist or dietician who is knowledgeable about WLS. A meal plan can then be implemented and your vitamin levels can also be checked frequently and supplemented if necessary.

- *You may need to educate your obstetrician and gynecologist:* Since WLS is a relatively recent type of surgery, many professionals don't know how to treat women who have had it.

- *Your risk of pregnancy complications drops, but doesn't go away:* Risks are reduced, but WLS patients still need monitoring for gestational diabetes.
- *You may face a body image battle:* Psychologically, a lot of women who have had surgery to lose weight have a very hard time accepting that they have to gain weight during pregnancy. Pregnancy can also be stressful, and people tend to eat when stressed. So women run the risk of going to extremes—either dieting while pregnant (which can have serious nutritional consequences for the baby), or gaining back some of the weight they lost because they are eating more food than they need due to stress.
- *You're more likely to have a caesarean:* Pregnant women who've had bariatric surgery are more likely to end up with a c-section, according to a 2004 study published in the *American Journal of Obstetrics and Gynecology.* It's not clear exactly why, and what factors are involved, but it helps to talk to your healthcare provider.

Pre-Op Tests

The pre-op tests that are required prior to WLS vary enormously from one provider to another and depend on your health status at the time of surgery, and often relate to any comorbidities you also have. These are usually performed by the provider but some may also be completed by your own MD.

Basic tests usually include weighing and recording, blood tests, blood pressure evaluation, oral glucose tolerance tests (if diabetic), EKGs, those relating to infection, and sleep studies, if necessary.

Some providers also insist on psychiatric assessment. You will be advised what this involves and whether there is any fasting required beforehand.

Preparing for Your Hospital Stay

While your hospital and bariatric team will give you a checklist of items to bring (or not bring) into your room when admitted for surgery, there are a few items that some patients recommend to make the stay a little more comfortable. Much will depend upon the surgery you are having and the duration of your stay but here are some suggestions.

- The most important are *medical documents and medications.* The latter with clear instructions for quantity and dosage attached.
- Some *money* (if allowed), but only for essentials—don't take items of special value since they could get lost or damaged.
- Some *baby or wet wipes* and/or facial cleansers for keeping yourself fresh and clean.
- *Lip balm* is a must to prevent your lips from cracking.
- An antiseptic *mouthwash* isn't essential but often welcome.
- An *eye mask* can be a godsend if you can't sleep in brightly lit conditions.
- *Ear plugs* are recommended since wards can be very noisy.
- Bottled sugar-free, flavored *water* as a nice change from the usual bedside jug of plain water.
- A *book* or *magazine* for some light reading—this probably isn't the best time to start *War and Peace* though!
- A *water spray* for spritzing the face and moistening the mouth and lips in the very early post-op hours when it's difficult to drink.
- A *phone charger* for your cell phone so that you can make those important calls home to family and friends who will need an update.
- *Headphones* if you intend to listen to music—hospital-provided ones (for their bed unit) can be uncomfortable.

- *A small padlock* for your case to secure any valuables, although it is far better to leave them at home.
- *An extra-large towel* for sleeping on. A flimsy cotton sheet over a plastic protector isn't the height of comfort so make yourself more snug with this improvised mattress topper.
- Some patients suffer post-op with trapped-gas pain. *Peppermint tea* helps, so pack a few teabags or consider packing an *antacid* to help.
- Loose-fitting *nightwear,* so you can recline comfortably.
- Your usual *toiletries*—some are usually provided, but they may not be as nice as your own.
- A *dressing gown* and *non-slip slippers*—for when you are back on your feet and on the move again.
- Your *CPAP machine* (the machine used to help breathing for people with sleep apnea) if you use one.
- Not essential, but sometimes a *back scratcher* and a small *hand-held fan* can make a big difference.
- A *small pillow* or cushion for placing between your body and seatbelt if traveling home by car.

After Surgery Pain Relief and Typical Care

Bariatric surgery is major surgery and, to varying degrees, it is normal to experience fatigue, nausea and vomiting, sleeplessness, surgical pain, weakness, light-headedness, gas pain and emotional ups and downs in the very early days and weeks after surgery.

Your comfort, however, is of the utmost importance to the surgical staff responsible for your care. So, although it is normal to experience some discomfort after surgery, keeping your pain under control is necessary for recovery and your team will do everything to facilitate this.

Generally, if you are feeling pain after surgery, you will be able to push a button on a cord to administer pain medication yourself. This is called "patient-controlled analgesia." The alternative is that the pain relief is administered to you by your care staff on a regular basis. As soon as you are able to tolerate fluids, your medical team will also add oral pain medication. You should be aware that you are not bothering staff if you ask for pain medicine. The sooner you are more comfortable, and are able to walk, breathe deeply, and cough, the sooner you will be on the road to complete recovery.

It helps to describe any pain you are experiencing to doctors and nurses on a scale—with 0 being no pain and 10 being the worst possible; or from none to mild, moderate, or severe. It also helps to plan ahead. If you are comfortable lying down, you may still need pain medication to get up and walk around, so request it if that is the case. Likewise, keep ahead of the pain—don't wait for the pain to be at its worst before you push the button or make a request. Pain medication works best when used to prevent pain. It should also be noted that the chances of becoming addicted to pain medicine are very low when it is used for a specific medical purpose, such as surgery.

Many patients sail through their surgery with little or minimal pain. Some feel a little at their incision site or as a result of the position their body was in during surgery. Some patients also experience neck and shoulder pain after laparoscopic bariatric surgery and gas pain from checking that internal closures are secure and non-leaking. All can be managed.

Following the advice of your team to change position, get on your feet, gradually breathe deeper, and exercise your feet and legs—this can make all the difference to your recovery and will certainly help to shorten your hospital stay.

Do, however, plan your recovery at home too. Think about your living environment and how you will manage after surgery. Are there many steps in your home? Is your bedroom upstairs? How accessible is the bathroom? Tell the bariatric staff in advance about this and they can help you make a home plan with your specific needs in mind. You might also want to enlist help from family or friends for your first few days at home.

Remember to keep in touch with your team and to attend all follow-up appointments that have been scheduled as part of your recovery. Also keep your primary care doctor informed of your progress and be sure to contact him or her with any medical concerns as well.

How Long Will I Be in the Hospital?

Depending on your procedure, how the surgery went, and your provider's individual preferences, you can expect to stay in the hospital for two to four nights, and longer if a complication occurs. You will only be discharged when the medical team is satisfied that you are fit to leave. Your provider will offer suggestions for activity, help needed, post-op injections, and other issues related to your post-op care.

Discharge Information and Incision Care

Most patients leave the hospital with discharge information to pass on to their MD and all medications required for immediate post-op care. This may include swabs for dealing with incisions and self-administered syringes for blood thinning for a number of days. Some will also have pain relief medications.

Most will also have instructions or arranged dates for follow-up appointments, or who and where to call to arrange for post-op checkups.

All patients should also have an emergency number and contact name in the unfortunate instance of a real emergency. Keep it safe and close by at all times.

Patients who have incisions will be instructed to keep their wound areas clean and dry, which means regular bathing and showering are off-limits (plus any swimming) until the wounds are fully healed.

Recovery—and When Can I Return to Work?

Most bariatric teams will encourage you to get active and mobile as soon as possible after surgery. Gentle and assisted walks in the hospital are encouraged along with bed or chair movement to help with recovery.

Once home, you need to rest but also still keep moving. By following good aftercare guidance, along these lines, you can expect to be returning to normal daily activities around two weeks post-op. Keyhole or laparascopic surgery helps with this quicker recovery as opposed to open surgery. However, this is a best-case scenario and you may well take longer to reach optimum recovery. Many take up to four weeks and some six weeks.

Regardless of case or timing it is crucial that you take sufficient time away from work and strenuous activity. Much will depend upon the type of job you have as to when it is considered safe to return—the average for a sedentary job-related worker is two to four weeks and, for those with a more strenuous physical role, four weeks plus.

It is important to take time away from the stresses and strains of everyday life to heal adequately and to refrain from engaging in physical activity that could cause internal injury.

Checkups

Upon leaving the hospital you will be given advice about the checkups you will need to have further down the line. These may well be with the surgeon but most likely be with a bariatric nurse and dietician. Some patients will also be checked for other comorbidities with their respective consultants—e.g., diabetic expert. Some will also meet with their mental health professional.

The schedule for this varies enormously and depends not just upon the provider but also upon the patient, their needs, their health history, and how they are coping after surgery.

These meetings and subsequent checkups are very important. Most checkup periods last for at least twelve months, the majority up to two years, and some others for three years. Privately funded patients are often given the option (for a price) to extend this after-care service.

When aftercare is deemed complete, the patient is then discharged and under the care of their own MD. Many can ask for a re-referral if a problem occurs after the usual aftercare period.

Blood tests for checking vitamin levels should still be carried out by the MD every six to twelve months, but again, this varies patient by patient.

At any time during aftercare if you have any causes for concern, contact your bariatric team, MD, or go to the emergency room for a real medical emergency.

Gastric Band Adjustment

The gastric band is an adjustable tool in WLS and therefore needs regulation, especially in the early stages after surgery. When the band is fuller, it causes more restriction and, when less full, allows food to move more quickly to the large stomach pouch.

Your very first fill doesn't happen until about four to six weeks after surgery, usually when you have started to eat solid foods again. The surgeon or specialist bariatric nurse will inject fluid into your band to cause restriction. This is done through an access port, which is just under the surface of your skin near your belly button. The procedure is simple and painless and only takes five to ten minutes. The extra restriction will bring about greater weight loss.

The aim with adjustment is to find a level at which there is sufficient restriction to bring about weight loss but not so tight that eating becomes an issue and nutritional needs are poorly met.

A patient can expect to have a number of fills and de-fills until this "sweet-spot" is found (or the Green Zone is reached, to coin another phrase).

Often after a "fill," the patient will need to adjust their diet for a few days to account for the new restriction. Many experts suggest that on the day of the "fill," you stick to fluids only, and then progress over the following two days to soft foods and then back onto solid foods.

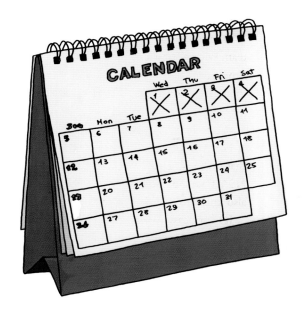

It is the wise patient who checks out an emergency number in case of any problems after a "fill," and if you intend to be away from home for any lengthy period, check if there are any facilities in the location you are staying. Ideally, don't schedule any adjustments just before you are due to travel.

You may need to get your band de-filled if you are sick and having trouble staying nourished and hydrated or have inflammation that causes problems. It is also possibly necessary if you become pregnant, although opinion divides on this.

Emergency ID Helpers

The wearing of an emergency bracelet, or medical ID band, after WLS, is something much discussed on forums. Check out your team's advice on this and then make up your own mind if you think it is necessary or not.

Bracelets and other jewelry or ID aids aside, there is a very real need for emergency services to know some valuable facts about you (and your surgery/allergies/next of kin) should you find yourself in an accident or in extreme difficulty.

One of the easiest ways is to provide the emergency team with what is called ICE ("In Case of Emergency") information. This information can mean the emergency services can contact your elected person (or persons) for help during an emergency. Don't underestimate the power of this.

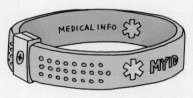

For example, my ICE contacts can tell any emergency operative that I have had an RNY Gastric Bypass and that I therefore cannot have Blind NG Tubing or NSAIDs. I am also sugar intolerant and have an allergy to Band-Aid adhesive. My contacts also know my GP's name and telephone number.

It's very easy to set up following the step-by-step guideline given online. Please do it today . . . none of us ever thinks it matters too much until it's an EMERGENCY!

Pre-Op Dietary Regimens

Almost all bariatric patients will be asked to follow a pre-operative or liver shrinkage diet prior to surgery. Many patients will query the validity of this, asking, "Why do I need to do it, and what if I can't adhere—I've failed at every other diet before!"

This is the special pre-operative diet that lasts for about two weeks (but sometimes longer) prior to weight loss surgery. After years of following and failing at diets, many patients understandably query their necessity. So are they necessary, and why?

This special pre-op diet is not necessarily a specific weight-reducing diet (although many patients will record weight loss while on it), but it has been designed to shrink the liver so that the surgeon can move it to one side to operate more easily and safely. It also increases the chances of surgery being performed laparoscopically (by keyhole). It's not an optional diet but a compulsory one and is only intended for before surgery. Some patients whose liver size is not significantly reduced will have their surgery aborted. This diet should not be followed after surgery or by anyone else.

Why Do I Need to Follow This Diet?

This diet is low in carbohydrate and fat. It will therefore reduce the glycogen (a form of sugar used for energy) stored in the liver. This results in the liver shrinking in size and softening.

When performing bariatric surgery laparoscopically, the surgeon will have to lift the liver to access the stomach. If the liver is heavy, fatty, and immobile, it is much more difficult for the surgeon to see and access the stomach. This could be a reason for changing to open surgery. Open surgery means a larger abdominal scar, which results in longer recovery and increased risks.

By following this diet, you are likely to lose weight before surgery but, more importantly, your liver will shrink, and you increase your chances of having a safe operation.

It is important to stick to the regimen you are given and for the stated time advised by your bariatric team. Don't be tempted to have a special or larger "last" meal the night before your surgery, as this will reverse the liver-reducing effects of the diet. If you feel like a last-ditch blow-out then have it before you start your pre-op diet!

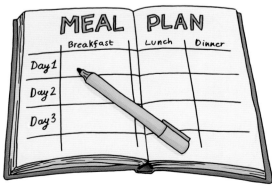

What Does the Diet Consist Of?

This very much depends upon your surgeon and your medical history. If you have diabetes, flag this to your team because you will need a different diet.

Some pre-op diets are principally "milk diets," where milk is the main foodstuff along with other fluids (like tea, coffee, and no-sugar flavored water), and a sugar-free Jello allowance.

Other diets that may be recommended are low-fat, carbohydrate-regulated (to about 100 g per day), and moderate in protein. Patients are given a diet sheet with recommendations of foods and their quantities. Both pre-op diets ask you to take a multivitamin and mineral tablet supplement every day.

It is possible that you will experience headaches or feel "light-headed" after starting this diet; this is quite usual and will pass in the first few days. This will prepare you for an important journey ahead—the start of something life-changing.

Post-Op Dietary Stages

Most bariatric surgeries have a staged reintroduction of eating after the surgery itself. At the simplest this is in three stages. These are

THE RED STAGE: the Fluids Stage—which is divided into Clear and Full Fluids

THE YELLOW STAGE: the Soft, Puréed, and Textured Stage

THE GREEN STAGE: Food for Life

Patients will be asked to gradually progress through these three stages with guidelines of the drinks and foods to ingest during this time, and with some guidance as to the time span in each. This process is much like weaning a baby and can't be hurried.

In the early stages, the fluids help with healing, whereas later, the softer textures prepare the pouch for food of a more solid consistency. There is no shortcut—a baby doesn't go from milk to a T-bone steak and a WLS patient won't either. There will also be huge differences among individuals, their surgeries, their tolerances, and, of course, their likes and dislikes. No one size fits all and it is fruitless to compare yourself with others at this juncture.

The Red Stage: Fluids

So you've had your surgery, returned from the hospital, and been given advice to continue with the staged reintroduction of food, beginning with fluids.

So what do they mean? Follow your surgeon's and bariatric team's advice to the letter (they will undoubtedly differ from one provider to another) but, in general, they will recommend clear then full fluids for just a few days after surgery, but sometimes for up to four weeks.

This is to minimize digestion, lessen the production of solid waste, and ensure maximum healing of your new gastrointestinal system.

WHAT ARE CLEAR FLUIDS?

These are fluids that you can see through and that will comfortably travel up a straw. They should be sipped slowly and never, ever gulped. It is important to have enough of them to keep hydrated, which means that you will almost constantly have one at your side in the very early days. Water is an obvious one but it is important to also have some "nutritional fluids" that will give you nourishment.

Below you will find a list of some choices, and I encourage you to experiment to find the ones you like and dislike. From experience, everything tastes strange and different at first, so keep experimenting and sampling so that boredom doesn't set in. Many fluids taste too sweet—so don't be afraid to dilute them to a more acceptable concentration and flavor (this is especially true with fruit juices).

The aim at this stage is to drink 10 to 15 cups (2.5–3.5 L) per day. This will be very hard to achieve at first, but do try. Spread them out evenly.

Everyone has different fluid requirements. The best way to check if you are well hydrated is to look at the color of your urine. If it's pale, you are drinking enough. If it's dark (straw-colored or darker) or if you produce little urine, you need to drink more.

Never have fizzy/carbonated drinks (see page 46 and 52).

Good Choices of Clear Fluids
- Water
- Tea—warm traditional, fruit, herbal teas
- Coffee—warm, ideally decaffeinated
- "No-added sugar" or "sugar-free" drinks
- Sugar-free Jello
- Chicken, beef, fish, or vegetable bouillon/ broth/consommé, or clear soup
- Whey protein isolate fruit drink (clear type), made with water
- Flavored sugar-free, non-carbonated water or protein water
- Sugar-free popsicles

These should be taken in addition to a daily multivitamin and calcium supplement.

It may seem like a long time, but it will only be a matter of days before you move on to full fluids. This stage provides a little more variety and nutrition to your regimen. This is a vital stage, since it prepares your surgically-altered stomach for more food. This stage can last just a few days, or a few weeks, according to surgical opinion.

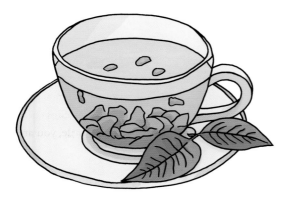

WHAT ARE FULL FLUIDS?
These are liquids that are considered smooth and pourable. Mix and match them with clear fluids for good hydration throughout the day. Taste and flavor may still be off, but variety is the key to moving sensibly through this stage and preparing your body for the next one. It does get better each and every day, and good habits can be quickly established at this stage to reap dividends further down the line.

Good Choices of Full Fluids
- Milk—skim, low-fat, soy, almond, rice, oat, and unsweetened nut varieties
- Milky chai-type tea—lightly spiced for added flavor
- Unsweetened plain yogurt without added sugar or fruit
- Smooth cream-style (but not high-fat) soups
- Whey protein isolate or other protein drinks that are low in fat and sugar—warm or cold and made with milk or water
- Mashed potato mixed with a little broth/ bouillon or gravy until thin and soup-like
- Diluted no-added-sugar fruit juice
- Tomato or vegetable juice—warm or chilled
- Homemade smoothies (not too thick), or store-bought, without added sugar and thinned with water
- "Diet" hot chocolate drinks without added sugar
- Smooth-style cup-a-soups
- Homemade vegetable, meat, and poultry soups that are puréed until smooth and diluted to a thin consistency
- Low-fat and low-sugar custards
- Very gently set egg custards

● Recipes suitable for this first stage of eating are color-coded RED.

Low-Fat Milk and Other "Skinny" Alternatives

Many pre-op and most post-op bariatric eating regimens encourage drinking low-fat milk for its nutritional benefits of good protein and high vitamin and mineral content. But there are many in the general population, and within the bariatric community, that find this a tall order. Some have lactose intolerance or insufficient lactase (the enzyme that is required to digest lactose, the natural sugar found in regular milk and dairy products) and suffer with bloating, gas, and changes in bowel habits.

Luckily there are a variety of delicious and nutrient-packed milk alternatives available for those with such intolerances or allergies. Take a look at the healthy and tasty options below but remember to choose and purchase unsweetened varieties to avoid excess sugar intake.

Soy Milk: This is made by soaking dry soy beans and grinding them with water and sometimes sugar. It's a good source of protein (about 7 g per 200 ml/7 fl ounces) and heart-healthy omega-3s. It is often fortified with calcium and vitamin D so that it compares favorably with cow's milk. You could opt for a light soy milk (with less fat and a lower calorie count), but remember it will have less protein in it, too.

Almond Milk: This is made from ground almonds and filtered water and, like soy milk, is fortified with calcium and vitamin D. It is a thin milk with a nutty taste and a great rich vitamin E content. The regular variety contains less protein than other milk alternatives (only about 1 g per 200 ml/7 fl ounces) but there is a protein-fortified version available which has 5 g per 200 ml/7 fl ounces, which may make a better choice if protein is your priority.

Rice Milk: This is a mixture of partially milled rice and water. Again, like almond milk, it has a thinner texture than ordinary milk but a sweeter flavor. Lower in protein at less than 1 g per 200 ml/7 fl ounces, it's a good choice for adding to breakfast cereals and in dessert recipes, providing you're meeting your protein needs with other foods.

Oat Milk: Made from oats and water, this milk has a sweet, earthy flavor. It's a good source of protein (about 4 g per 200 ml/7 fl ounces) and is fortified with calcium, vitamin A, and vitamin D. Oat milk generally has a higher sugar profile than other milk alternatives due to its natural starch content.

Hemp Milk: This alternative is made from hemp seeds that have been soaked, then ground with water, to make a creamy milk with a nutty taste. It has a moderate amount of protein (about 2 g per 200 ml/7 fl ounces) but is a great source of essential fatty acids and powerful antioxidants.

Coconut Milk: This is milk made from the grated meat of the coconut, usually fortified with vitamin A and D. It usually has 1 g protein per 200 ml/7 fl ounces and has a higher saturated fat level than other milk alternatives. It does, however, have a good creamy texture and a distinctive tropical flavor, which works well with some recipes, but not with all.

The Yellow Stage: Soft Foods

If you don't experience any problems with Stage 1: Fluids (the Red Stage) then you will quickly move on to the second stage, which incorporates smooth, puréed, soft, mashable, textured, and then crispy food. This is typically called the Soft Food Stage (the Yellow Stage).

This stage is typically followed for about two to six weeks after surgery, but always follow your bariatric team's advice as to when to start it and when to move on.

This stage mirrors the weaning stages of a baby from milk to solid food, so don't be in a hurry to whizz through it or become disheartened with setbacks.

Start slowly and make sure that initially your food choices are soft and loose—first-stage smooth baby-food texture is what you are aiming for here. Progress to foods that can be easily crushed or mashed with a fork or mixed to a "slurry" with milk, gravy, or sauce. Don't be put off when something doesn't suit or settle well . . . try it again a few days later. You'll find that some days some foods go down easily and comfortably and the next day they don't. Learn to listen to your body and its signals of satisfaction or upset.

You will still need to be aiming for at least 2 liters (about 8 glasses) of liquid a day in addition to these small "meals." Don't drink twenty minutes before, twenty minutes after, or during a meal, and aim for four to six "meals" per day.

Eat slowly and as soon as you are full or experience something akin to "fullness," STOP EATING. Just one extra mouthful or teaspoonful at this stage can send your system into overload and—there is no pleasant way of saying this—what went down will either come back up or make you feel very uncomfortable. Remember your new stomach pouch is only about the size of an egg.

You may find it convenient to freeze soft meals for this stage—a stash stored away in the freezer in an ice-cube tray can be helpful for those times you don't feel like making something from scratch. Don't go overboard, since you won't be eating very much and a monotonous round of the same meal-flavors isn't good for morale.

Below are some good food choices for this stage—introduce them gradually and then replace as time goes on with ones that have more texture and flavor.

Aim to have three small "meals" a day (of a ramekin or small saucer size), along with your fluids.

Crispy foods, which melt or dissolve into bits in water, such as Melba toast, crispbreads, crackers, and breadsticks, can also be introduced in the latter stages of this second stage. Chew them very thoroughly until they are reduced to a smooth paste in your mouth. Don't mistake these for crunchy foods, like fruit, salad, and crisp vegetables, which would cause problems at this stage.

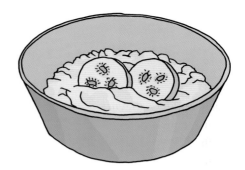

This is ideally the time when you should start looking at preparing your own bariatric-friendly soft food meals from scratch. Many processed and ready-made alternatives have hidden sugars and fats to make them taste good which can be a problem for the bariatric. Venture into the new world of bariatric cooking and take control for the best outcome. Just a few recipes to begin with will bring huge dividends. Learn to decipher information on food labels (see page 64) so that you are well-armed when shopping.

When looking at such foods, you are aiming for low-fat (about less than 3 g fat per 100 g listed) and sugars (not carbs) of under 5 g per 100 g. A quick tip here is that fat has 3 letters (so 3 percent) and sugar has 5 (so 5 percent). Remember this is per 100 g, not per portion.

As for sugar, toleration levels vary enormously. Many bypass patients can't tolerate more than 7 to 12 g sugar in any one portion size or they experience "dumping syndrome" (see page 40).

Good Choices of Soft Foods

- Shredded wheat, porridge, or oats with plenty of low-fat milk to make a runny consistency
- Mashed banana with a little yogurt
- Very softly cooked scrambled egg
- Finely ground or puréed chicken or turkey in gravy
- Puréed fish in a thin sauce
- Puréed canned fish (tuna, sardines, salmon, or mackerel) in a thin tomato sauce
- Soft and smooth low-fat pâté or spread
- Plain low-fat cottage cheese
- Puréed mashed potato with thin gravy
- Puréed canned and very tender boiled vegetables, such as carrot and cauliflower
- Low-fat and low-sugar fromage frais and thinned quark
- Light and smooth low-fat and low-sugar mousse made with milk
- Warmed mashed potato mixed with grated low-fat cheese or light cream/soft cheese
- Milky pudding, such as rice or tapioca, without too much added sugar
- Puréed cauliflower in a low-fat cheese sauce
- Puréed, thickened, or soft piece vegetable and chicken soups
- Puréed casseroles and stews of a thinnish consistency
- Very gently cooked and soft plain omelet
- Poached or soft-boiled egg
- Soft beans, lentils, and peas, puréed or mashed for a little texture
- Thick fruit smoothies
- Puréed avocado
- Small portions of home-cooked or ready-prepared and puréed main dishes like shepherd's pie, fish in sauce, mild chili, casseroles, or their vegetarian alternatives
- Low-sugar sorbets, frozen yogurts, and low-sugar and low-fat ice creams
- Silken or smooth tofu
- Crispy foods like crispbreads, breadsticks, Melba toast, and crackers

These should be taken in addition to a daily multivitamin and calcium supplement.

Recipes suitable for this second stage of eating are color-coded YELLOW.

Emergency Supplies Box

I believe things go wrong when you're not prepared. You know what I mean . . . when there's been a traffic accident and all exits are closed, so you have to wait to move on; when you're on the road and all you see are fast-food signs; when you arrive somewhere late and there's nothing on the menu that's suitable for you; and when you're dashing between activities or work appointments and there isn't the ideal "food-to-go." I've been there and now have an emergency supply box in the trunk of my car to cope with all these situations . . . sometimes it has been a lifesaver, when poor weather has tripled my journey time!

You might want to consider putting the following in your emergency box:
- water, plain or flavored, but not carbonated
- a low-fat and low-sugar cereal bar or protein bar
- a small packet of mixed unsalted nuts or soy beans
- a small packet of protein chips
- a small jar of low-fat pâté or paste in a jar with crackers (don't forget a small knife for spreading)
- a low-fat and low-sugar protein drink (ideally ready-to-drink or in a shakeable flask)
- a small bag of mixed seeds
- a small packet of olives
- a "healthy" low-fat and low-GI snack or meal-cup that just needs boiling water to rehydrate
- a small packet of dried fruit
- a screwtop jar or keep-fresh container with a little bariatric-friendly cereal and a couple of long-life mini cartons of milk
- a small packet of beef jerky
- a couple of sugar-free candies or mints
- low-fat snacks like rice cakes, crackers, crispbreads, or Melba toast.

If you're not in the habit of taking your medications with you, pack a single dose for those unexpected times when you might be seriously delayed.

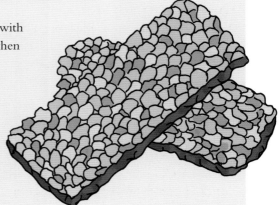

The Green Stage: Food for Life

Only when you have been able to tolerate a variety of the foods in Stage 2 should you then move on to Stage 3. This stage, which we call Food For Life—but others call "normal food" or "regular food"—typically occurs between eight to sixteen weeks post-op and is a transitionary stage, in which you progress through to the kind of foods that you will eat for the rest of your life.

The timing of this stage varies enormously and you should always follow the advice of your bariatric team as to the best time to proceed. This is the point at which you should be able to try to eat a variety of solid food, albeit in small amounts. Try using a small side plate, children's plate, salad plate, or bariatric portion plate as a guideline for serving size and proportions (see page 63). This is the time at which you get a glimpse into what the future holds and what you are likely to be eating from now on.

Foods to begin with should have a soft and moist texture so may have to be served with a little sauce, salsa, dressing, or gravy, so they form a moist mouthful; although, as time goes on, a drier texture is encouraged for constriction and an ideal transition through the newly altered digestive system.

These so-called "slider" foods help in the early days but can mean that you are able to digest more at a later stage just when you are looking for "satiety" and don't want foods to pass through the stomach or pouch too quickly. Gradually cut down on them as you progress from week to week so that they don't hamper your progress (see page 46).

This is not a diet with a beginning and an end, nor is there need for a rush to get to your "goal weight." Take it slowly, learn to recognize when you are full and satisfied, and don't eat beyond that point of satisfaction. As time goes on, gastric bypass and sleeve patients will learn to recognize this point and gastric band patients will certainly, in time, find their "sweet spot."

It makes good sense to cook meals for everyone in the family rather than separate ones at this point. Why be a slave to a new regimen that will not happily suit everyone? Everyone can benefit from the foods here: high-protein, low-fat, and low-sugar. Add an extra accompaniment for those growing members of the family or a sweet treat from time to time to get an ideal balance.

THE REGIMEN AND SOME RULES

- *High-protein, low-fat, and low-sugar* is the mantra.
- Always eat your *protein first* (the meat, poultry, eggs, fish) on your plate, then move onto the vegetables and fruit, and finally the carbohydrate element—potatoes, rice, pasta.
- Choose *lean protein* with any visible fat removed (e.g., chicken skin); aim for *low-fat* (you won't always manage it, but aim for less than 3 g fat per 100 g); and always opt for a *low-sugar* version of a meal (the syndrome known as "dumping"—see page 40—is thought to occur when you eat more than 7 to 15 g of sugar in one serving).
- Eat *three meals per day* with a couple of small snacks if necessary. These should satisfy you. But beware of developing a "grazing" eating pattern of small snacks throughout the day.
- *Eat healthy,* solid food. Soft food undoubtedly slips down more easily, but you can end up eating more over the course of the day. If your food is drier and more solid, you will generally eat less overall and stay fuller for longer.

LOW-SUGAR

- *Eat slowly* and stop as soon as you feel full. Take tiny bites and chew each piece 10 to 25 times. Chew, chew, chew, and chew some more! Once you feel full, STOP! Gone are the days when you need to clear your plate.

- *Keep your fluid intake up.* It is also a good idea not to drink immediately before, during, or after a meal (see the 20:20:20 rule on page 70) so that your stomach isn't full from fluids. Get into this habit as soon as you can.

- Take your *multivitamin, calcium, and other supplements* every day religiously . . . they will ensure that you have the best chance of getting all the additional nutrition you require that may not be supplied from the reduced amount of food you are eating.

- The hardest nutrient to keep on track with is undoubtedly *protein*. Aim for 70 g per day. Quite difficult to begin with and do consider a protein whey isolate powder if you consistently fall short. A portion of this powder in food or drink can quickly and efficiently provide 25 g or a third of your requirements in one fell swoop (or scoop)!

● Recipes suitable for this 3rd and final stage of eating are color-coded GREEN. You can of course also have those color-coded Red and Yellow, too.

Substitutions for Cream

Whether it's a spoonful in your coffee, a dollop on your dessert, or ingredient in sauce, cream is often used as a base for many different dishes. However, despite its versatility, cream is calorie-dense and lacks significant nutrients. One tablespoon of heavy cream packs about 50 calories and 5 grams of fat. Whether you're trying to cut calories or simply don't have cream on hand, there are many different alternatives that can take the place of this heavy cooking staple.

Easy Substitutions: If you're simply in a pinch and are lacking cream in your refrigerator, there are many quick and easy substitutions that will give you a similar flavor and texture. Switching to reduced-fat yogurt or sour cream can cut calories down substantially per serving and reduce fat. For recipes that require thickening, mix 2 tablespoons cornstarch with 1 cup (250 ml) milk, low-fat cream, or crème fraîche, and allow the mixture to thicken before adding to recipes.

Fat-free half-and-half in your morning coffee can also provide a healthier alternative to cream, containing only 20 calories and no fat in 2 tablespoons. In addition to coffee, fat-free half-and-half can also be incorporated into sauces and soups to achieve the desired creamy texture without the extra calories.

Soft Tofu: Tofu offers versatility as a non-dairy alternative to cream. Depending on the type that you purchase, it can be used to achieve many different consistencies in your dish. Soft tofu will yield a lighter cream, whereas extra-firm tofu will produce a thicker one. Puréed tofu can be used in a 1:1 ratio in place of heavy cream as a much healthier and lower-fat option.

Coconut Milk: Coconut milk is a flavorful substitute for cream, suitable for vegans, and an excellent option for those with lactose intolerance. Much like tofu, coconut milk is available in different consistencies and also as full-fat or reduced-fat. It also provides some essential nutrients that cream lacks, such as vitamin C and iron. Due to its naturally sweet flavor, coconut milk works best as a substitute in Thai dishes such as curries, and in ice cream and other desserts.

Greek Yogurt and Quark: Greek yogurt, which is lower in fat and high in protein, provides another great substitute for heavy cream. Simply add a little water or milk to achieve a similar consistency to cream. While the reduced fat content in Greek yogurt creates a much healthier alternative, when used in baked goods, it tends to create a finished product that is more dense and moist. For the best results, substitute full-fat Greek yogurt in place of a low-fat or fat-free variety. You can also try mixing Greek yogurt with whole or 2% milk to contribute more richness and flavor. In addition, because yogurt does not hold up to heat in quite the same way as cream, it is important to use a lower heat when making sauces or soups. Too much heat too fast can curdle the yogurt, creating a less than ideal final product. Quark, a low-fat skim milk product can be used pretty much in the same way as Greek yogurt. There are both plain and flavored varieties to choose from, such as lemon, raspberry, and vanilla.

Eggs: Eggs provide a lower-fat and easy last-resort substitute. For each ¼ cup (60 ml) serving of cream, add one whole egg or two egg whites. Before adding them to your recipe, beat the eggs until they are creamy and then fold them in. Using eggs as a substitute lends similar thickening properties as cream but works best when baking desserts and sauces.

Whether it's a lighter indulgence or a quick fix that you're looking for, there are a variety of products and combinations that can take the place of cream. By using items that may already be on-hand in your kitchen, you can create anything from a creamy sauce to a frozen dessert, all while saving yourself some extra calories.

Basics of the Bariatric Diet

Bariatric Eating: It's Not Just About Eating Less

Losing and keeping the pounds off after WLS largely depends not just on eating less, but also upon eating the right foods, with the right nutrition, in the right amounts. But finding the foods you can and want to eat, and making the transition from your "old life" to a healthy new one can be challenging. Even if you know a great deal about nutrition, putting this into practice is hard.

From the early post-op days on Fluids and Soft Foods, moving onto "Food for Life," it is important to practice "mindful eating," making sure that you eat right with every bite, as much as you can.

This can often be easier in the early "honeymoon" stage after surgery, when you might not have any real appetite or hunger for food, than in the later stages, though there is a danger of not eating or drinking enough. During this time, you can maximize your weight loss results by eating right and exercising regularly.

Protein will be your greatest priority during this time, and it is fair to say will always be. Most patients are told to aim for 70 g per day to facilitate good health and healing.

Carbohydrates come next, and although these vary by surgical procedure as well as medical issues (like diabetes); 130 g per day is often what is quoted in bariatric surgery scientific literature. The aim here is to ingest many of these as complex carbs, found in plant-based foods, rather than simple sugars. This figure may sound overwhelming and most likely won't happen in the first few months after surgery, but it is certainly something to aim for at least six to nine months post-op. Gastric bypass patients will also have to watch sugars for fear of "dumping syndrome." Aim for under 5 g sugar (not carbs) per 100 g—I rarely have a dish with more than 7 to 10 g sugar per serving to reduce this risk.

Fats, often mistakenly labeled the "bad guys," also have a place, but this varies enormously according to procedure, and the mantra here is to steer clear of too many saturated fats, keeping the level down to under 3 g fat per 100 g.

Add to that the advice about eating "five-a-day" and keeping up the fiber; hydrating well with at least 2 liters (8 glasses) of water; not forgetting the daily taking of multivitamins, calcium, and other supplements; and you have a regimen that can be more than a little testing.

It has been my challenge as a food writer to develop recipes for all these stages of post-op eating, taking some of the guesswork out of cooking on a daily basis. The recipes in this book have all been devised and tested to not only work (a minimum requirement!) but to also adhere to these nutritional guidelines and to be deliciously tasty, too. Some are very simple and will not test even the most inexperienced cook, and others will offer ideas for those who like to experiment and entertain. All have been considered carefully in terms of cost, seasonality, and cuisine to offer the virtues of variety. They also have been devised to suit the needs and appetites of everyone so that mealtimes can be a pleasant experience with family and friends.

The recipes have been classified with the traffic-light coded system as suitable for the Red (Fluids) Stage; the Yellow (Soft Foods) Stage; and finally the Green (Food for Life) Stage, to guide a patient on the journey of eating well again. People's tolerances vary greatly; so while these recipes may be recommended as being appropriate for a specific stage, only the patient will know for sure when they can best be tolerated.

Each recipe also has a nutritional analysis breakdown so that you can keep a check on the calories, protein, carbohydrates, and fat. Used in conjunction with a food tracker, you can see how your levels are working out over a day and week.

But recipes are one thing and general eating is another. I would still advocate that patients become avid, if not fanatical, food label readers (see how to on page 64). Understand and be aware that food manufacturers add sugar, salt, and fat to foods to make them taste better. Check out the best nutritional options—take a little extra time in the supermarket to find them; speak to other bariatrics on websites and forums for advice; and pass on anything you find at support groups for everyone to benefit.

What have I learned since my own surgery? Well, that I have a new regimen to follow. I have forgotten about dieting and the old destructive starve and binge ways of old. I now have a diet, but I'm not on a diet. This took some time to get right. I followed the three stages of eating after surgery in a relaxed way. I considered myself to be weaning rather like a baby and realized that some days some things worked, and other days they didn't. But I always did retry and, as a result, my diet has great variety.

MINDFUL EATING

I have learned to practice "mindful" eating—trying to eat only when hungry, not when bored, sad, or angry. I eat slowly and savor every mouthful and I chew, chew, and then chew some more. I have quite easily slipped into a healthy daily regimen of three meals and two snacks. I also sit at the table to eat with a knife and fork without distractions. No more sitting on the sofa with a packet of something or other, watching TV, and then wondering who ate all the goodies a little while later!

I have also adhered to the advice given to me by my dietician about not grazing, and to ease up as time has gone by with sloppy/slider foods that won't help me feel full for long. And, (this has come as a surprise) I have started to move much more. I have found the best exercise for me is the one that I will do. So I walk, dance, swim, and occasionally hit the gym.

Some of my tips for success include cooking for one to serve two. If I didn't, my husband would eat one-and-a-half portions and be sitting on the gainers bench, well away from me on the losers. I also use a smaller plate and sometimes bariatric cutlery (to slow down my pace of eating) so that portion control is more manageable. I use a bariatric portion plate to help with this so that I not only get the food choice right but also in the correct proportions for a bariatric.

I plan for emergencies by having bariatric-friendly food in the freezer and a couple of snacks in the trunk of my car should I get caught in traffic or be running very late. In restaurants (which I visit at least twice a week), I tend to order two starters instead of a starter and main course and am not shy about ordering off a children's menu or asking for a "doggy bag" to take home something I can't finish. I often "upcycle" or repurpose these leftovers into something quite different from the original.

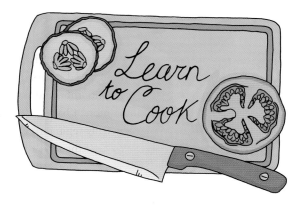

However, the best advice I can give has been left until the end: *Learn to cook*—that way you can control your food intake, know just what you are eating, and still have a good, healthy relationship with food. This doesn't mean being a slave to the kitchen—there are lots of healthy convenient foods out there to make life easier—just try to avoid the unhealthy ready-made and junk-food varieties.

Eat Right with Every Bite

This was my mantra at the beginning of my WLS journey and something I adhered to stringently for the first eighteen months post-op. It's now something I aspire to, recognizing that "real life" isn't about perfection but progress. I still work hard on making protein my priority at every meal, keeping fats at a sensible level, eating more complex than simple carbs, hydrating well, and taking my vitamins and supplements daily. But I also recognize that joy comes from the occasional treat, the planned indulgence, and sometimes practicing self-love and forgiveness when it goes a tad off-track.

What I do know is that there isn't a situation that can't be turned around, so I accept rather than fight some of them. I then get back on track or back to basics (see page 80), and restore good habits whenever I know that they are in danger of being hijacked.

Trust me when I say that this will in all likelihood happen to you, too, but it doesn't mean throwing in the towel—it's just life! This book mirrors some of the questions I have asked over the years about bariatric eating (and nourishment by association), and it should arm you with resolve and solutions for when those times come.

The Question of Calories: Should You Count?

"How many calories should I be eating?" is perhaps the most popular question asked by post-op patients.

Each and every time I'm asked, I say that I don't count them because my own surgeon and dietician told me I didn't need to. I just had to look at the quality of the food I was eating (along with some effective portion-control), so I could forget the old diet mentality.

What joy! Because DIET for me often meant "Dare I Eat This?" And yet this query persists within the WLS community. It's the reason I still give calorie counts on my recipes, because so many complain if I don't. We seem to be swayed to the point of hysteria by nutritional stats.

But don't just take it from me. Read the advice below from a reputable bariatric surgery provider who answers the question and backs it up with some facts and figures.

CALORIE COUNTING AFTER BARIATRIC SURGERY

There's lots of information online around what and how much you should eat after bariatric surgery. Many patients come across this while researching surgical options, and it is often very confusing. One of the questions asked most often is: How many calories should I be having each day after my surgery?

Unfortunately the answer to this question is not clear-cut. At present there is not a validated predictive equation for estimating calorie requirements for patients after bariatric surgery. Therefore, any calorie targets that you have read about online are not based on robust scientific evidence. Furthermore, your calorie intake will change as the months go by after surgery. Your portion sizes will begin to increase.

Each patient's food intake after surgery should be more focused on the qualitative as opposed to the quantitative. You will want to know how you are doing identifying your new hunger and satiety cues, what types of food you are choosing, in what settings you are eating your meals (social occasions or eating out), and any challenges you may have. There should be far less interest in the number of calories.

Below I will discuss some of the reasons why calorie counting is not useful after surgery, and what you can monitor for yourself instead.

A SHIFT AWAY FROM THE "DIETING MENTALITY"

Many patients have understandably developed a strong habit of counting calories after many, many years of dieting. After your surgery, focus on changing this mentality and setting up healthy eating habits and thoughts around food. It is this that is going to set you up for long-term success and help to prevent relapses. Counting calories will not help, but it will cause you much more stress and anxiety!

BARIATRIC SURGERY IS NOT A DIET. IT IS A LIFE-LONG CHANGE

As you all already know, bariatric surgery is not a short-term solution—it is a long-term solution for the rest of your life. Therefore, the focus is on life-long positive habits. At the end of the day, counting calories is just another fad diet. No one wants to keep tabs on the calories in each of their meals for the rest of their life, and nor should you want to!

FOOD QUALITY

Bariatric surgery reduces the amount of food you are physically able to eat, but it has no effect on the nutritional quality of the food you eat. Calorie counting does not help here either, as the lowest calorie choices are not always the most nutritious.

WHAT SHOULD I FOCUS ON WITH MY DIET AFTER SURGERY?

- Eat regular meals.
- Listen to your hunger and satiety cues and eat accordingly.
- Focus on protein and low-starch vegetables at meal times and then fruit and dairy as snacks if you have the appetite.
- Keep carbohydrates to a minimum and choose low GI, whole grain options when you do have them (such as brown basmati rice instead of white rice).
- Keep hydrated and remember to drink.
- Take your daily supplements.
- Exercise as appropriate for you.
- Keep up regular contact with your bariatric team. That is why they are there, so you do not have to figure out things on your own!
- And remember, always quality over quantity!

Many patients are concerned about the small portions of food they are eating immediately after surgery, and start counting calories to keep tabs on their nutrition. These small portions are only short term, and this is one of the reasons doctors do your pre-surgery blood tests—so they can begin to correct any nutritional deficiencies prior to surgery.

Keeping up your supplements during this time is also critical to achieve adequate nutrition. This is why your team keeps in such close contact during the first few months, so they can make sure you are choosing the right types of foods.

Protein the Priority and Protein Supplements

During all your pre-op (and post-op) discussions with your bariatric team you will have been advised that protein is your priority post-op. It is the single most important dietary consideration—without it you will experience muscle wasting, hair loss, and weakness after WLS. But it's not easy, and it can be tricky to get a high level of protein in your diet in the early days after WLS, when your appetite is low.

You will undoubtedly be encouraged to get protein from the food you consume but also may be advised to look at protein supplements if you're falling short or want to ensure from the onset that you are meeting your daily protein requirements. Some people who have trouble achieving the recommended levels opt to take a protein drink supplement. There are many available in a multitude of flavors, but if you're considering one, choose one that is low in fat, sugar, and calories. Don't opt for the bodybuilder's version!

Others boost their protein levels by adding dried skim milk or unflavored protein powder to their food. Tasteless and virtually unnoticeable, it can be stirred into soups, stews, smoothie-type drinks, and most puréed foods for a welcome protein boost.

WHY IS PROTEIN IMPORTANT?

Proteins are a part of every cell, tissue, and organ in our bodies. These body proteins are constantly being broken down and replaced. The body does not store protein for later use, so consuming adequate high quality protein is necessary, otherwise the body will suffer. When protein intake is not adequate, the body will break down lean body mass to compensate. Loss of lean body mass is inevitable for WLS patients or other individuals following a very low-calorie diet. To minimize that loss, sufficient high-quality protein must be consumed.

When you step into a health food store or a vitamin shop, there is often an abundance of protein supplements to choose from and sales people, claiming they are "nutritionists," trying to sell you the best liquid or powder protein products on the market. There is a large assortment of protein supplementation available to consumers; however, it is essential to recognize that some supplements are of higher quality than others. For WLS patients, it can be very confusing if you are not aware of what to look for when it comes to protein supplementation.

WHEN SHOULD LIQUID OR POWDER PROTEIN SUPPLEMENTS BE USED?

There is a huge divide between providers who promote the use of protein supplements and those who do not after WLS. Take the advice of your own team—they know you and are responsible for your care.

For those WLS patients who are recommended protein supplements, the choice is vast. If you are constantly under-scoring on your protein tally, they often make a viable alternative.

WHAT IS THE BEST-QUALITY LIQUID OR POWDER PROTEIN SUPPLEMENT?

Commercial protein supplements are available in many flavors, textures, tastes, and prices; however, the product's amino acid composition is of the most importance when choosing protein supplements. Amino acids are the building blocks of protein. There are nine indispensable (essential) amino acids (IAA) and eleven dispensable (nonessential) amino acids (DAA). The IAA must come from dietary intake because the body is incapable of producing these compounds.

During rapid weight loss, when protein supplements are the main source of dietary protein intake, it is essential to choose products that contain all of the IAA. It is important when choosing protein supplements that they have a score of 100 on the protein digestibility corrected amino acid score (PDCAAS). This is a system that was developed as a method to evaluate protein quality. PDCAAS scores of as close to 100 as possible are desired to indicate that the protein supplement contains the appropriate amount of IAA that the body needs.

Protein supplements that are made from whey, casein, soy, and egg whites have a PDCAA score of 100. It is important to recognize that many of these protein sources are sold as either concentrates or isolates.

ISOLATES

In general, isolates tend to have a higher concentration of protein than concentrate forms. For whey protein isolates, the filtration process removes a lot of the lactose, minerals, and fat in the product; therefore, these products have very little or no lactose, and often provide more protein in smaller volumes. These products may be beneficial to patients who have lactose intolerance. Also, isolates tend to have a better mixability and a cleaner taste, therefore compliance is often better with these products.

CONCENTRATES

Whey protein concentrates have a lower concentration of protein and higher concentration of lactose. Although the protein is of good quality, the percentage of protein will vary. Consumers can always view the nutrition label for accurate protein quantities.

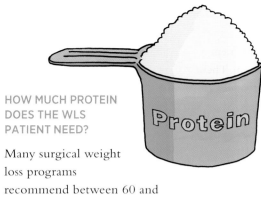

HOW MUCH PROTEIN DOES THE WLS PATIENT NEED?

Many surgical weight loss programs recommend between 60 and 80 grams of protein per day for the adjustable gastric band (AGB), vertical sleeve gastrectomy (VSG), and the Roux-en-Y gastric bypass (RYGB). The biliopancreatic diversion with duodenal switch (BPD/DS) requires approximately 90 grams of protein per day to accommodate for the malabsorption associated with this procedure, and sometimes more.

These recommendations are for individuals without complications (malabsorptive procedures alter digestion, thus causing the food to be poorly digested and incompletely absorbed). Those with complications will have different protein needs. The exact requirements for postoperative WLS patients with complications are not defined. It is recommended to follow up with your surgeon and dietician to assess protein requirements and adequate protein intake.

PROTEIN SUPPLEMENTS AND MEAL REPLACEMENT SHAKES: THEY ARE DIFFERENT

It is important to also recognize that there is a difference between protein supplements and meal replacement shakes. Many meal replacement supplements often have a blend of soy, casein, or whey protein to enhance the texture or taste of the product. Meal replacement shakes also have higher amounts of vitamins and minerals and varying amounts of carbohydrates and fiber.

One thing to consider is that meal replacement shakes are often designed to supplement a diet that includes animal and plant protein. These should not be used as the sole source of protein or calories in the diet for an extended period of time.

WHAT PROTEIN SUPPLEMENTS SHOULD BE AVOIDED?

Collagen-based protein supplements are not a good source of high-quality protein and should not be used as the sole source of protein intake. Collagen-based protein supplements do not contain all of the indispensable amino acids that the body needs. When consuming collagen-based products as your sole source of protein, loss of lean body mass can occur, even if you are meeting your daily protein goals.

DO WLS PATIENTS NEED LIQUID OR POWDER PROTEIN SUPPLEMENTS FOR LIFE?

As you begin to consume more food after surgery, the need for protein supplementation often declines or ceases. Relying solely on protein supplements to meet your protein needs is not recommended after the early post-operative liquid stage. Foods of high biological value are encouraged (meat, poultry, fish, eggs, milk). However, WLS patients who cannot meet their protein needs from food alone may benefit from supplementation of high-quality protein.

WHAT ARE THE DANGERS OF EXCESSIVE PROTEIN INTAKE?

If you are not well hydrated, excessive protein intake may contribute to dehydration. It is also important to remember that additional protein intake, above the recommended amount, may inhibit the consumption of other important nutrients.

The Question of Caffeine

Many bariatric teams recommend limiting or avoiding caffeine after WLS. Caffeine reduces your body's ability to absorb nutrients like iron and calcium, and the acidity of many caffeinated beverages can irritate the stomach and increase your risk of acid reflux and heartburn. Therefore take your team's advice before consuming.

Caffeine can be found in
- green and black tea
- coffee
- hot chocolate
- energy drinks
- chocolate and foods that contain it.

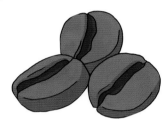

Be Savvy About Sugar

Many doctors and scientists are increasingly concerned that sugar may be more of a culprit in the obesity epidemic than fat. Why? The energy boost it provides is rapidly followed by a slump as the rapid rise in blood sugar is counteracted by insulin in the body. This causes a sudden drop in blood sugar which then has you reaching for more sugary foods to create that energy high again. So you end up eating more. Sugar is contributing to tooth decay and dental pain in around a third of adults and children, too. And more and more evidence is linking high sugar intake to problems like heart disease, cancer, liver disease, and even Alzheimer's disease and dementia.

Reducing sugar intake in any way will help gradually wean your body off the sweet stuff and reduce your cravings, breaking that addictive cycle that will make ditching sugar easier in the long run. It's so important that the World Health Organization has recommended that we eat no

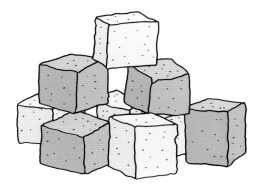

more than 6 teaspoons (24 g) of sugar a day, hidden sugar included. That includes all sugar—including honey, fruit sugar, maple syrup—apart from the sugar found in milk or in whole fruit and vegetables.

If you are able to go completely cold turkey, be reassured that it doesn't take long for the body to readjust to being sugar-free and those cravings DO diminish. And you will soon notice the improvements in your health, mood, and weight!

HOW DO YOU CUT BACK ON SUGAR?

- Cutting out the added sugar in the obvious culprits—hot drinks, desserts, or candy—is a great place to start.
- Check the labels of processed foods to find how many grams of hidden sugar they contain.
- Ditch the fizzy drinks (which, as WLS patients, we shouldn't imbibe anyway) which can contain 9 teaspoons of sugar or more.
- Don't forget fruit juice. Even a 7 fl ounce–glass (200 ml) of orange juice contains 5 teaspoons of sugar—and some smoothies can contain many more.
- Watch out for breakfast cereal. Besides the "chocolate-filled" options, even the "healthy" granola-type dried fruit cereal can also contain high sugar levels.
- Careful in the coffee shops. The latte with a muffin can pack a hefty sugar and calorie count.
- Step back from the sweeteners. So-called "natural sweeteners" like honey and fruit juice are still sugars and count towards your

6 teaspoons (24 g) a day limit. "Sugar-free" may mean packed with artificial sweeteners, which are not a great choice for life-long nutrition. While some may be healthier than sugar and can even protect against tooth decay, the long-term effects of sweeteners are not well-known. Besides, they do nothing to reduce your desire for that sugary fix. Instead, you need to reduce your sweet tooth overall. If you slowly reduce your need for that intense sweetness, you can reduce your sugar intake without really noticing—without the use of chemicals.

Dumping Syndrome

WHAT IS IT?

This lovely-sounding syndrome results from the rapid passage (or dumping) of undigested food into the small intestine, causing a rapid shift of fluid as the body tries to "dilute" the contents of the intestine. This shift in fluid causes cramping and diarrhea and can also result in a drop in blood pressure, causing weakness and sweating.

WHY DOES A GASTRIC BYPASS MAKE THIS POSSIBLE?

As a result of the surgery, you no longer have the valve that regulates how quickly food empties out of the stomach. The surgery also causes food to enter the gastrointestinal tract at a point lower down than it's supposed to due to the first part of the small intestine having been "bypassed."

Sugar consumption is also the biggest cause of "dumping" for many gastric bypass patients (and some others too). Controlling the amount of sugar you have, depending upon sensitivity, is therefore critical if you don't want to experience some pretty awful symptoms.

That first part of the small intestine is where sugars normally are metabolized. So basically you're now dumping sugar lower in the intestines, where they aren't equipped to handle it. The result: your body rebels! So dumping happens when food (especially sugar) moves too quickly though the stomach and is "dumped" into the small intestine. The body has a tough time handling this rapid "dumping" and responds by adding a large amount of fluid to the small intestine. This fluid is the cause of patient dumping symptoms. Thankfully, this does not usually require medical treatment.

Translation: Eat the wrong thing and you can feel really, really sick for many hours.

Here's one patient's account of what dumping syndrome feels like.

Shortly after eating a food my body doesn't tolerate (sugar, milk, sugary milk products, or starchy carbs) I begin to feel a bit disoriented and dizzy, and then an overall sense of confusion or panic takes over my mind and body. This is a mild state of delirium. Then I begin sweating. Profuse sweating that can completely soak my hair, my clothes; it drips and glistens on my skin. During this state of sweaty panic I feel like I'm out of my mind! A few times during extremely dramatic dumping episodes I literally thought I was dying, the state of distress was that severe.

CAUSES OF DUMPING SYNDROME

- Eating candies or foods high in sugar
- Eating too much at one meal
- Having solids and fluids together
- Eating foods that are fried, fatty, or greasy

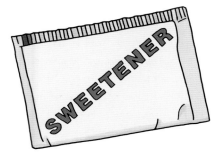

HOW TO AVOID DUMPING SYNDROME

- Avoid/limit concentrated sugars, like those in cookies, cakes, pies, sugar, and syrup.
- Read food labels for sugar content. Avoid foods with sugar listed among the first three ingredients.
- Eat six small meals daily instead of three large meals if you are very susceptible.
- Eat slowly.
- Avoid eating and drinking at the same time. Wait twenty minutes before and after a meal to drink fluids. Drink low-sugar beverages only.

A Note about Sugar

"Sugar Free" foods and drinks often contain sugar alcohols which may not be well tolerated either. So note: Words ending in "-ose" are generally forms of sugar.

The following is a list of sugars and sugar alcohols to try to avoid in large quantities:

barley malt	lactose
brown sugar	lactitol
cane sugar	levulose
confectioners' sugar	maltose
corn syrup	mannitol
corn sweeteners	maple syrup
dextrose	molasses
fructose	raw sugar
glucose	sorghum
granulated sugar	sucrose
honey	sorbitol
high fructose corn syrup	turbinado
invert sugar	table sugar
isomalt	xylitol

While dumping syndrome is certainly no fun to experience, the negative feedback is often a convincing motivator to stick to your post–weight loss surgery diet guidelines. If you'd always wished your dentist could have just pulled out that "sweet tooth," this could be the next best thing.

I've had patient after patient tell me how their addiction to sugar was instantly broken after experiencing dumping syndrome. In truth, it sounds bad and feels worse.

TYPES OF DUMPING SYNDROME

There are two kinds of dumping: early and late. Both occur after a meal, especially after eating foods high in fat, carbohydrates, or sugar (both table and natural, like that found in fruit).

Early dumping occurs within thirty minutes of eating a meal. In addition to high fat, high carbohydrate, and high sugar foods, it can also be brought on by eating foods that are too hot or too cold, or drinking liquids during your meal. Such early symptoms include bloating, vomiting, diarrhea, heart palpitations, nausea, sweating, dizziness, and a rapid heart rate.

Late dumping is a form of hypoglycemia (low blood sugar). When you ingest too much sugar, your now-smaller stomach does not digest it properly, so your intestines absorb and deposit too much of it into your bloodstream. Your body then compensates by releasing more insulin which makes your blood sugar drop. Symptoms for this late dumping include anxiety, heart palpitations, fainting, fatigue, diarrhea, rapid heart rate, a strong feeling of hunger, sweating, weakness, dizziness, and confusion.

As long as you do not stray from your prescribed bariatric diet, you should not experience "dumping syndrome." For this reason, many patients view it as a "blessing in disguise" since it helps them to keep their diet on track.

Interestingly, some patients' tolerance for foods that might trigger "dumping syndrome" can change over time. Some find that several years out of surgery they can tolerate small amounts of foods they could not eat in the earlier days.

As many as 80 percent of gastric bypass patients experience "dumping syndrome" but less than 5 percent have serious problems with it. As a general rule, the more of your stomach that has been removed, the more likely you are to dump.

The treatment is to wait and let the symptoms pass—many patients find bed rest helpful.

IS IT A "HYPO" OR DUMPING SYNDROME?

Some patients who have had bypass surgery experience what they think are "dumping syndrome" symptoms but confusingly are not— they can be episodes of reactive hypoglycemia. They are similar in terms of symptoms but need quite different treatment to alleviate.

WHAT IS REACTIVE HYPOGLYCEMIA?

Reactive hypoglycemia (non-insulinoma pancreatogenous hypoglycemia syndrome) is a seemingly rare and potentially serious complication following gastric bypass.

Normal glucose levels are between 4.4 to 6.1 mmol/L (82 to 110 mg/dL). The brain can only use glucose to function. If the blood glucose level falls too low, the brain cannot function. Diabetics who inject themselves with too much insulin can develop reactive hypoglycemia because insulin drops their blood glucose to very low levels. Low blood glucose levels can occur in certain patients after gastric bypass and this can produce several symptoms of varied severity from mild to severe.

HOW DO I FIND OUT IF I HAVE IT?

If you think you may have low blood sugar after eating, you should measure your blood sugar level using a glucometer, available at any pharmacy. Do the test an hour before a meal, a few minutes after eating, an hour afterward, two hours after, and so on. Keep a food log and keep track of your blood glucose readings at all the various times before and after meals. Also track your symptoms and your glucose levels during these symptoms.

If your blood glucose is less than 4 mmol/L (<82 mg/dL) at any one of these measurements, please call your bariatric team or MD for a follow-up visit. Bring the results you recorded with you.

HOW IS REACTIVE HYPOGLYCEMIA TREATED?

You and your bariatric team need to understand what's going on with your body. Your food log—including the times you eat, and any blood sugar highs or lows on that same log—will be used to spot any patterns that might develop. Over time you'll be able to spot trends and understand how your body is working a bit better.

Reactive hypoglycemia is manageable. Make sure you are following your dietary guidelines and instructions—eat protein first, then the complex carbohydrates, and lastly healthy fats.

You will need to experiment with foods and figure out what *your* triggers are, and what are the foods that work *best* to bring you back from a sugar crash.

Many published experiments show why you should not treat those with reactive hypoglycemia like diabetes. For example, diabetics are asked to eat sweets to bring their blood sugar up quickly from an overdose of insulin (the cause of their hypoglycemia).

That doesn't work well in reactive hypoglycemia post-gastric bypass. It will just cause a new cycle of crashes and sugar spikes.

You need a *balance* of nutrients, not sugar. For most patients, peanut butter crackers, a handful of grapes and a slice of cheese, or a granola bar works best. The rule of thumb is to take a bit of simple carbohydrates to bring the crash up quickly, then a balance of protein and fat to keep the glucose up. When out of the house, carry a granola bar for emergencies.

In cases of severe hypoglycemia with loss of consciousness, immediate treatment with 3 to 4 glucose tablets (5 g each) or 3 to 4 teaspoons of honey should be given to patients who can swallow. If no response, call emergency services.

Dear Diary: Keeping a Journal

As so many successful dieters can attest, if you want to succeed at losing weight, it helps to pay attention not only to what you eat but also to what you write. As you follow your new WLS regimen, writing down what you put into your mouth each day may help keep you from overeating, or from eating the wrong things.

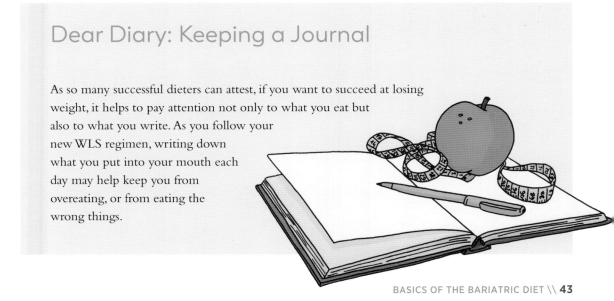

In fact, the National Weight Control Registry, a well-regarded, long-term weight loss study, found that journaling is one of the most powerful tools used by people who have lost weight and kept it off. Here are four more reasons to start a food diary or journal today:

You'll be more aware of mindless eating.

What did you eat yesterday? Sure, you can remember your meals, but what about those mindless between-meal nibbles or snacks that you grazed on? The WLS regimen recommends a protein- and fiber-rich mid-morning and mid-afternoon snack if you need it, but it's often easy to overlook the other little bites you may inadvertently indulge in throughout the day. And they can add up. Writing everything down will help you become more aware of your previously unacknowledged eating habits.

You'll discover your diet detours.

Are you a late-night refrigerator raider? Do you find yourself hitting the vending machine to beat mid-afternoon fatigue at the office because you forgot to bring healthy snacks with you? Do you indulge in sweets when you're unhappy, stressed, or even, paradoxically, when you're especially happy? Knowing what your eating triggers are will help keep you on track. To break bad habits, you should record not only what and when you eat but also the circumstances that prompted you to overindulge and make those unhealthy choices in the first place.

You'll see your progress at a glance.

If you're committed to losing weight and improving your health, your food diary will give you a glimpse at the progress you're making. Just compare entries from week to week. If you're staying on track, you'll note a downturn in refined carbs, sugars, and unhealthy fats and see an uptick in healthier options, including heart-healthy vegetables, fruits, and whole grains. Simply seeing all those smart food choices at a glance will be positive reinforcement as you work toward your health and weight loss goals.

I've made it easy for you.

All of the recipes in this book have nutritional analyses with them so that you can see quickly the protein, carbs, fat, and ideal WLS portion. If you use it with a journal or diary to log your foods and track your progress it makes analysis easy. You can also jot down your thoughts and feelings, sort through challenges you've faced, and record your successes.

But I'm a Vegetarian or Vegan

Does being a vegetarian have any special impact on the consideration of weight loss surgery? Are the restrictions of such a diet (or way of life) going to prove too problematic for those who elect for surgery?

The good news, that comes off the back of a recent study at the University of Oxford, is that a well-planned vegetarian or vegan diet is most apt for the weight loss surgery patient. Indeed the risks (such as hospitalization and death from heart disease) are 32 percent lower in vegetarians than in people who choose to eat meat and fish. Researchers say that the health benefits that are often experienced by vegetarians are likely related to having lower blood pressure and cholesterol levels.

It has long been noted that decreasing your intake of saturated fat and cholesterol has a positive impact on such health issues. The increase of heart-healthy unsaturated fats that are part of a typical healthy vegetarian diet may have the edge over a carnivorous one.

The secret, of course, is making sure that the vegetarian or vegan diet is a healthy, varied, and nutritious one. A vegetarian diet excludes meat, poultry, fish, and seafood. A vegan diet additionally excludes eggs and dairy. These foods are typical and staple protein sources for patients who have had weight loss surgery . . . so what to have instead?

Well, thankfully, there are a wide variety of plant-based protein sources from which to choose. These include beans, lentils, nuts, tofu, soy, and quinoa. They can also be supplemented with vegan cheeses, and yogurt, as well as plant-based egg substitutes.

Cooking from scratch and preparing your own vegetarian meals is undoubtedly better than buying ready-prepared special dishes, but there are some good vegetarian staples like veggie burgers, vegetable roasts, and casseroles out there in the supermarket aisles.

It is wise to carefully plan (with a registered dietician) your post-op vegetarian or vegan diet to ensure adequate protein intake. Since plant-based foods are often less protein-dense than their animal-based counterparts, some vegetarian and vegan WLS patients may need to consider including some protein supplements (like drinks, bars, and powders) in their diet to meet the average daily goal of about 70 g of protein a day.

Cautionary and Warning Foods

Possible Problematic Foods

There are some cautionary solid foods that may give rise to problems both long and short term after WLS. Somewhat surprisingly, some of these appear to be tolerated one day and then prove problematic the next. Often, foods become easier to tolerate further out from surgery, but as with all things, there are exceptions to the rule.

Ask a group of WLS patients for these and the list will prove almost endless, which goes to show that one person's tolerability to foods is not another's.

Many dieticians say to proceed with caution with the following foods:

- no caution; just a straight NO to fizzy drinks for life
- many say no to chewing gum in case of swallowing and provoking blockages
- non-toasted bread, especially soft, white bread, which turns to the consistency of wallpaper paste when thoroughly chewed and sits uncomfortably in the pouch
- tough and fibrous meat that has a very chewy texture from tougher cuts of meat, chops, and steaks
- overcooked rice and pasta, which becomes very glutinous
- stringy vegetables, such as green beans
- pineapple, mushrooms, and corn, which have a toughened texture

- seeds and edible skins that come from fruits and vegetables
- dried fruits that have a high concentrated sugar content
- some granulated sweeteners—even the calorie-free ones—which can provoke "dumping syndrome."

Slider Foods

To the WLS patient, slider foods are the bane of good intentions and ignorance, often causing dumping syndrome, weight loss plateaus, and eventually weight gain. Slider foods, to WLS patients, are soft, simple, processed carbohydrates of little or no nutritional value that slide right through the surgical stomach pouch without providing nutrition or satiation. The most innocent of slider foods are crackers, often eaten with warm tea or other beverages, to soothe the stomach in illness or while recovering from surgery.

UNDERSTANDING SLIDER FOODS

The most commonly consumed slider foods include pretzels, crackers (saltines, graham, Ritz), filled cracker snacks (such as Ritz Bits), popcorn, cheese snacks (Cheetos) or cheese crackers, tortilla chips with salsa, potato chips, sugar-free cookies, cakes, and candy. You will notice these slider foods are often salty and cause a dry mouth, so they must be ingested with liquid to be

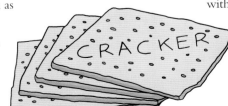

palatable. This is how they become slider foods. They are also, most often, void of nutritional value.

For WLS patients, the process of digestion is different than those who have not undergone gastric surgery. When slider foods are consumed, they go into the stomach pouch and exit directly into the jejunum, where the simple carbohydrate slurry is quickly absorbed and stored by the body. There is little thermic effect in the digestion of simple carbohydrates like there is in the digestion of protein, so little metabolic energy is expended. In most cases, patients who eat slider foods will experience a weight loss plateau and possibly the setback of weight gain. And sadly, they will begin to believe their surgical stomach pouch is not functioning properly because they never feel fullness or restriction like they experience when eating protein.

The very nature of the surgical gastric pouch is to cause feelings of tightness when one has eaten enough food. However, when soft, simple carbohydrates are eaten, this tightness does not result and one can continue to eat unmeasured, copious amounts of non-nutritional food without ever feeling uncomfortable.

Many patients turn to slider foods for this very reason. They do not like the discomfort that results when the pouch is full from eating a measured portion of lean animal or dairy protein without liquids. Yet it is this very restriction that is the desired result of the surgery. The discomfort is intended to signal the cessation of eating. Remembering the "Protein First" rule is crucial to weight management with bariatric surgery.

Gastric bypass, gastric banding (lap-band), and gastric sleeve patients are instructed to follow a high protein diet to facilitate healing and promote weight loss. Bariatric centers and bariatric teams advise what is commonly known among weight loss surgery patients as the "Four Rules," the most important of which is "Protein First." That means of all nutrients and food groups (protein, veggies, complex carbohydrates, then fat and alcohol) the patient is required to eat protein first.

Protein is not always the most comfortable food choice for weight loss surgery patients who feel restriction after eating a very small amount of food. However, for the surgical tool to work correctly, a diet rich in protein and low in simple carbohydrate slider foods must be observed. The high-protein diet must be followed even after a healthy body weight has been achieved in order to maintain a healthy weight and avoid weight regain.

WLS and Flatulence

A sensitive subject after WLS but nonetheless one that crops up every now and again relates to gas post-op. Not just the increased occurrence after WLS but the associated bad smell that also accompanies it for so many patients.

Why does it occur? Is there anything one can do about it, diet-wise? And are there any solutions for controlling and dealing with it?

Many patients note some change in the amount, timing, and character of their flatus after surgery. Usually, this is a temporary issue, but it can be quite concerning. Severe malabsorptive procedures such as duodenal switch or distal gastric bypass are more frequently associated with complaints.

Changing dietary intake is certainly one of the major causes of altered flatus or flatulence (which comes out of your bottom), as opposed to borborygmus (burping). Certain foods result in more sulphur compounds in the gas and create a worse smell. Carbonation is usually absorbed into the bloodstream, and the body will expel a fair amount of it via your exhaled breath. The altered bowel motility and absorption as a result of weight loss surgery also can result in more or smellier gas.

Noise associated with gas can be from the abdomen (bowel sounds) or with the passage of gas through the anus (or an ostomy). While the buttock can make some noise, most is from the internal sphincter.

STRATEGIES TO REDUCE AMOUNT, ODOR, OR CONTROL THE TIMING OF FLATULENCE

Gastroesophageal Reflux Disease (GERD). If you have a history of GERD/esophageal reflux, you likely swallow air frequently without noticing, as you swallow to clear acid from your esophagus, even away from meals. Avoid gum chewing or other oral fixations that may increase this habit. With weight loss, and as an effect of a smaller stomach, the actual reflux and pain are usually better, but the behavior often persists. Swallowed nitrogen gas is the largest single component of most flatus.

Do Not Eat Too Fast. Most of us have accelerated motility in the small bowel. Food already gets to the colon (large bowel) quickly, and fast eating may get it there more quickly. The bacteria in the colon will have more fuel to form gas if you are dumping undigested food into their home.

Do Not Eat Too Much. This is especially true for many who are partially lactose intolerant. A little more food can be fine, but too many extra bites can really cause havoc. Also, overeating can be a stimulus to accelerated bowel motility and "dumping" (see page 40).

Avoid Your Trigger Foods. The most common complaint about flatulence is with additional dietary fiber for constipation. A few people also find alcohol or lactose bad, and almost anyone will have a threshold of sorbitol (a non-digestible sugar) of no more than a few grams a day. Rice is supposed to be one of the safest foods to not cause gas, so consider that when cooking or ordering a meal. Also, probiotic yogurt may be useful for irritable bowel symptoms in some and has little risk.

Privacy. This may sound obvious, but, if you can, go for a walk or find privacy before releasing gas.

Medication/Supplements. Consider an intestinal deodorant containing bismuth subgallate (Devrom is an example). You can also try antacids, but be careful and discuss this with your surgeon and dietician. Seek medical attention if you have severe or persistent associated symptoms.

Social Interactions in the Workplace. If you know your work colleagues well, try bringing up the subject politely with them. They will often appreciate it and less fuss may well be made when a "bad moment" occurs.

Out and About. On an airplane, use a fleece sweater as cushion. At the gym, look for cardio machines near the fan or vent, and remember extra effort can cause uncontrolled gas-release when you lift weights.

Remember, part of what makes us laugh about this is the social discomfort we all have with gas. Again, the most important message is to give your body and gut time to adapt. The first year after weight loss surgery is often very different from later years, and some real change occurs in the ability of the gut to absorb nutrients at various locations.

Medications After WLS

Many people with obesity have severe health problems such as diabetes, high blood pressure, elevated cholesterol, and coronary heart disease. Patients who undergo bariatric surgery and successfully lose weight see these health conditions improve, and they may be able to stop some medications with their doctor's advice.

Taking fewer prescription medications doesn't always mean no more pills, though. Good health is the goal, not fewer pills. Many people actually take more pills, as they follow vitamin and mineral plans, and have better awareness of the benefits.

What Effect Does Weight Loss Surgery Have on Medications?

Prescription or over-the-counter drugs may be absorbed differently after surgery, depending on the type of procedure. Your medication therapy may be affected by this change. In the early period right after surgery, larger tablets or capsules may not be recommended by your surgeon, so that pills do not become stuck. Because of this, your surgeon may recommend that you take your medications in a different form, such as crushed, liquid, suspension, chewable, sublingual, or injectable. Some long-acting medications and "enteric coated" medication may not be crushable. Some medication may be crushed and administered with food.

Sleeve gastrectomy and adjustable gastric banding tend to cause little to no change in the absorption of medications. Roux-en-Y gastric bypass and duodenal switch can have more significant changes in how medications are absorbed. Check with your surgeon and pharmacist about how you should take each of your medications. Some patients need a higher dose of antidepressants to produce the same effect. This is not a complication, but you need to be aware of how you feel and speak up with all your caregivers.

Will my medications change after bariatric surgery? Maybe. Some doses may change. Some medication doses may decrease as the obesity-related health conditions improve. For example, diabetic patients often require less insulin after surgery because glucose control can improve quickly. Patients who take high blood pressure and cholesterol medication can see their doses lowered if these disease states improve. Any changes in prescription medication should be overseen by your doctor; this is not something that you should do yourself.

Which medications should I avoid after weight loss surgery? Your surgeon or bariatric physician can offer guidance on this topic.

DON'T TAKE! One clear class of medications to avoid after Roux-en-Y gastric bypass is the "non-steroidal anti-inflammatory drugs" (NSAIDs), which can cause ulcers or stomach irritation in anyone but are especially linked to a kind of ulcer called "marginal ulcer," after gastric bypass. Marginal ulcers can bleed or perforate. Usually they are not fatal, but they can cause months or years of misery, and are a common cause of re-operation and even (rarely) reversal of gastric bypass.

Some surgeons advise limiting the use of NSAIDs after sleeve gastrectomy and adjustable gastric banding. Corticosteroids (such as prednisone) can also cause ulcers and poor healing but may be necessary in some situations. Some long-acting, extended-release, or enteric-coated medications may not be absorbed as well after bariatric surgery, so it is important that you work with your surgeon and primary care physician to monitor how well your medications are working. Your doctor may choose an immediate-release medication in some cases if the concern is high enough. Finally, some prescription medications can be associated with weight gain, so you and your doctor can consider the risk of weight gain versus the benefit of that medication. There may be alternative medications in some cases with less weight gain as a side effect.

Are there any additional prescription medications I will have to take after bariatric surgery? Some patients may require antacid medications, either temporarily or indefinitely. Some surgeons prescribe a temporary medication for gallstone prevention if you still have a gallbladder. Ask your surgeon if these will be needed.

Are all medications crushable? Not all medications are crushable. Whether or not a medication can be crushed depends on the drug formulation. In general, uncoated, immediate-release tablets may be crushed. It is important that you are VERY careful with medications, so please always check with your surgeon, primary physician, or pharmacist prior to making medication decisions.

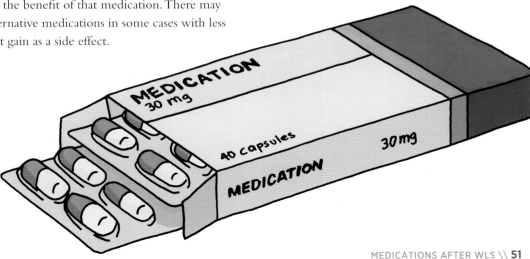

Fluids and Hydration for Life

Getting enough hydration after surgery is probably the first hurdle any WLS patient needs to tackle. Water allows your body to heal, transport nutrients, rid itself of toxins, maintain blood pressure, regulate body temperature and many more essential but minor things. Dehydration—mild or severe—needs addressing from the onset.

At its mildest, dehydration can lead to headaches, cramping, sleepiness, and general poor concentration—at its worst it can be life-threatening. For your body to function at its best, you must constantly replace any fluids lost by taking in more through beverages and foods.

In general, you will be advised to aim for 8 servings of 8 fl ounces (250 ml), more if the weather is warm. This is a tall order when you are told not to drink twenty minutes either side of a meal or during it. If you do consume food and liquid together, you risk stretching your stoma (in the case of a gastric band); your pouch (in the case of a gastric bypass); or your sleeve (with sleeve gastrectomy).

Water will undoubtedly be your best friend but you can also consider well-diluted low-sugar drinks; low-fat milk, tea, and coffee; diluted fruit juice; popsicles; and bariatric-friendly protein drinks and waters.

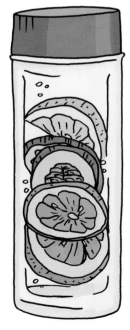

Of course you can also take in fluids with your foods. Fruits, fish, eggs, salads, and vegetables also have a high fluid content.

Avoid fizzy drinks, as these can cause bloating and, in severe cases, can help stretch the new pouch. Likewise, don't use a straw because it will only allow you to take in more air, which can make you feel bloated.

Meeting your needs for fluids isn't easy but try

- setting your timer, phone, or alarm at regular intervals to remind you to drink
- measuring out your daily requirement into bottles or cups, or make a checklist of them and check off each time you complete one
- keeping a bottle or sipping cup alongside you at all times—by your desk, on the kitchen counter, in the car, in your exercise bag.

Water: The Essential Ingredient

The original zero-calorie drink, water is cheap, available almost everywhere, and an important part of a healthy lifestyle, especially for bariatrics. Many people find it hard to drink water, after many years of soft drinks, sodas, and juice. Here are some tips to help you increase you water intake.

- *Temperature:* Find out which water temperature you like the most, and make sure you always have some on hand. If you enjoy your water ice cold, find a container where you can keep it iced all day.

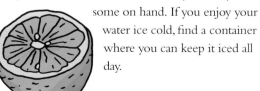

- *Flavor:* Add lemon juice, lime juice, orange slices, cucumber slices, berries, herbs or herb extracts (like peppermint).
- *Bubbles:* Are a no-no. If you like sodas, it's important to wean yourself off them. For reasons why, see page 46.
- *Bottles:* Having a water bottle you like around you all the time will make you want to fill it up over and over, ensuring you get as much as you need. BPA-free, of course.
- *Straws:* Avoid if you can, since you'll simply fill your reduced stomach/pouch with air before it has the chance to enjoy the water.
- *Wake Up with Water:* Starting your day with a glass of water is easier because you're thirsty from that (hopefully) nice long night of sleep you've had. Warm water can help to relax a tight pouch especially for those who have a band.
- *Brew Something:* Sometimes we overlook tea as a source of hydration, but without too much caffeine and sugar, tea is a great hydrator.
- *Remember How Good It Is:* Once you start a healthy water habit, you'll start realizing how good you feel when you do drink water. And if you start losing weight, keep that in mind every time you think about drinking something else.
- *Use It as a Diet Tool:* Before you reach for a snack, drink a glass of water. Before you eat, and in between meals, feelings of thirst can be mistaken for feelings of hunger. Drink more water and save calories when you're really just thirsty.
- *Keep It Clean:* Tap water is usually fine, but sometimes water and even ice can get a strange flavor that makes you not want to drink it. So invest in a water filter, water filtration system, water softener, or water delivery. Anything that helps your water taste better is an investment worth making.

Alcohol: To Drink or Not to Drink?

This is a thorny question within the bariatric community—with some saying go ahead, some being cautionary, and others advising against.

Alcohol provides calories and little other nutrition or other important nutrients, but it does have social importance for many.

The general advice is that you don't consider alcohol for the first six months (as a minimum) after surgery and then stay within the recommendations of a daily maximum (usually one drink for women and two for men), and that you 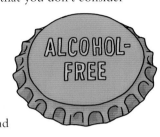 don't use it to replace a meal. Also, do not drink alcohol with your food or choose a soda mixer with spirits. If you really do feel cornered with this, swirl the mixture to remove as much gas as possible.

Drinking alcohol can so easily derail all good intentions because it relaxes you, meaning you don't always stick to what you had planned and are at risk of eating high-calorie foods. There is also the danger of risky behavior when inhibitions are lowered.

And since the alcohol seems to be absorbed so much faster than with the non-WLS patient, the bloodstream will quickly show a rise in alcohol content—so driving is most certainly not advised after imbibing.

More important for some has been the increased incidence of cross-addiction with alcohol after WLS. If you feel alcohol is becoming a problem post-op, then you are strongly urged to ask for help.

Vital Vitamins and Nutritional Supplements

Guidelines and Formulations

Regardless of your surgery type, your bariatric team will advise on taking a multivitamin and maybe some other supplements for the rest of your life. Why? Well, first of all, you're eating far less. Before your surgery, you were able to eat larger quantities of food, so you were probably getting most of the vitamins and minerals you needed from the food you ate. Now, with your smaller stomach pouch, you're undoubtedly eating less and so cannot get all the nutrients you require from your daily food intake.

If you also underwent one of the malabsorptive surgeries (like the Roux-en-Y gastric bypass, for example), you're also not absorbing your vitamins and nutrients from food as efficiently as before, so an additional reason to reinforce the need for a regular daily supplement and long-term regimen.

Your own bariatric team will advise you specifically on what you individually need so always follow their advice to the letter, however here is the general advice:

MULTIVITAMINS AND SUPPLEMENTS AFTER A GASTRIC BAND

With this type of surgery, you do not have altered absorption of nutrients, so, if you are following a healthy diet, you should not become deficient in any vitamins and minerals. You will get most of your calcium requirements if you have three portions of dairy food in your diet each day (one portion = 7 fl ounces/200 ml milk, a matchbox-size piece of cheese, or 1 cup/225 g of yogurt, for example). However, while you are losing weight, you might like to take one multivitamin tablet daily, and perhaps a calcium supplement, if meeting your requirements with dairy foods proves too challenging. Choose ones that can be broken up into smaller pieces to swallow so that they do not become stuck in your band stoma. Alternatively, choose a chewable or liquid version, but avoid the capsule formulations. You might also want to ask your pharmacist about any existing medication you take to see if it's available in liquid form.

MULTIVITAMINS AND SUPPLEMENTS AFTER A GASTRIC BYPASS

After a gastric bypass, it is very important to take additional vitamins as you are no longer able to absorb sufficient amounts of them from your food. Vitamin and mineral deficiency is an avoidable complication. Unfortunately, vitamin levels are hard to detect accurately in the body and you could become deficient before you show signs or symptoms. As always, prevention is better than cure. Undoubtedly, the best source of vitamins and minerals is a healthy diet, so eat mindfully with a good variety of foods.

Most bariatric teams recommend a multivitamin tablet and a calcium supplement daily. Sometimes, additional iron may be prescribed if your routine blood tests show you are becoming anemic. You can choose chewable or liquid versions.

MULTIVITAMINS AND SUPPLEMENTS AFTER A GASTRIC SLEEVE

Most bariatric teams recommend the same vitamin and mineral regimen as gastric bypass patients, even though the surgery is different. See above.

MULTIVITAMINS AND SUPPLEMENTS AFTER A DUODENAL SWITCH

Advice here is similar to that for gastric bypass patients but, because there is a greater degree of malabsorption, you may have to watch your protein intake and your uptake of vitamins A, D, E, and K, as well as iron and zinc. Most dieticians will recommend that you try to eat double the amount of protein usually recommended to compensate for this. In addition, you will need to take a multivitamin tablet daily. This will cover many of the essential vitamins and minerals but there are others which you need to pay special attention to in addition to this. A and D are very important fat-soluble vitamins, and because you are not absorbing fats you will need to take a water soluble version. Many people take ADEK vitamins (generally three per day) to maintain a proper level. Calcium is the most important mineral to take after duodenal switch surgery. You must take about 1,500 to 2,000 mg per day, ideally in the form of calcium citrate (rather than calcium carbonate which is not so easily absorbed). Many duodenal switch patients are also prescribed potassium straight after surgery, but do not need it as time progresses. About 10 percent of patients will also need to take iron but your MD or bariatric team will advise if this is necessary.

TIPS

- Do not take your multivitamin and calcium supplement at the same time or the nutrients will not be absorbed properly.
- Avoid taking any vitamins and supplements with caffeine as this can interfere with absorption.
- Take your vitamins and supplements at the same time every day—once this becomes a habit, you'll be less likely to forget taking them.
- Take your vitamins between meals—remember that your stomach pouch is small, if you take them before, with liquid, you won't be able to eat as much food as you need to.

GOOD CHOICES

It is important to select high-quality vitamin and mineral supplements that your body can absorb well. There are a good number of products available—just make sure that they contain both vitamins and minerals.

It is possible to download the latest guidelines for requirements—check against those for the best option. You may be one of the fortunate ones where your MD or insurance provider will supply and pay for your supplements, although in many areas this is now generally falling under the remit of patients themselves (often after two years of aftercare), so your choice may well be limited with what prescription you are given.

There are also now a good range of specially formulated bariatric vitamins and supplements that have been produced specifically for WLS patients. Some are in tablet and capsule form, others as chewable tablets, more as a dissolvable drink, and a few as a powder or chew. Some can be purchased via the internet (and can be automatically reordered for you) taking the guesswork out of complying with this lifelong need.

Feeling Tired?
Check Your Vitamin B12

Are you feeling more than tired? Been getting enough sleep, nourishment, and exercise? Then it might be worth looking at your vitamin B12 intake.

B12 deficiency has been called sneaky and harmful, with serious health consequences. One reason is that B12 levels are not typically checked in a routine blood screening and the symptoms can be missed because they mimic a number of other diseases. As a WLS patient, ensure that you are tested. Some patients will be advised to have a regular injection.

Certain groups of people may be at risk for developing a B12 deficiency. Among them are strict vegetarians or vegans who eat no animal foods whatsoever, people over fifty, people taking diabetic or acid-suppressing drugs, and those who have had their digestive systems altered. People who undergo WLS procedures such as gastric bypass and sleeve gastrectomy face a significantly increased risk of B12 and other nutrient deficiencies.

Signs of B12 deficiency include fatigue, lethargy, incontinence, tingling of fingers and toes, shortness of breath, forgetfulness, confusion, and depression.

Fortunately, there are many ways to ensure that you are getting enough B12. It is an essential water-soluble vitamin that is found in animal foods, such as shellfish, eggs, and meat. Additionally, B12 can be taken as a supplement. The daily recommended amount of vitamin B12 is 2.4 micrograms (mcg) per day, although people over fifty may require more.

Cooked clams and beef liver are particularly rich sources of vitamin B12. Other good sources include fish, meat, poultry, eggs, milk, and milk products such as yogurt and cheese. For vegetarians, many breakfast cereals are fortified with vitamin B12 that can be readily absorbed and utilized.

Aim to use food first, but if you have experienced bariatric surgery, discuss the use of a dietary supplement as part of your post-surgical follow-up routine. There are many good oral spray ones available, or consider a regular injection via your MD or bariatric team.

Stocking Up on the Best Ingredients

Your bariatric cupboard, refrigerator, and freezer may not look very different post-op to pre-op, save for the fact that they may have less food inside, look bare of junk food, and hopefully will have healthier choices on the shelves.

There's no doubt that most of the time fresh is best, but there are also some great frozen, dried, and canned options that will suit everyday cooking. This is a great time for experimentation, and hopefully you will be tempted to try out some new foods, different options, and recommendations in this book and from other WLS patients.

Manufacturers are constantly producing new lines, and several specialized health food producers have now started to launch lines for either the WLS patient or the food regimen they follow. High-protein foods are enjoying a heyday at the moment, alongside lower-fat and reduced-sugar alternatives.

A hard and fast list wouldn't be enormously helpful since these foods are introduced and withdrawn at alarming speed, but keep an eye out for new foods to try to bring variety to your regimen.

Most WLS patients find that alongside their usual fresh ingredients they like to keep an array of canned and jarred foods such as beans, tomatoes, olives, soups, milks, fish, pickles, vinegars, and herbs and spices. Lentils, rice, Jello, nuts, crispbreads, pasta, oats, sweeteners, cereals, and grains are also most useful, and a well-stocked refrigerator with chilled deli meats, cheese, yogurt, eggs, spreads, and dips doesn't go amiss.

The freezer can become a valuable ally if stocked with fish, ground meats, poultry, shellfish, meat portions, and frozen fruit.

Learning to cook and trying out new food ideas means that you can control your food intake, know just what you are eating, and still have a good healthy relationship with food.

Smart Shopping Tips and Bargains for Smaller Appetites

It's a well-known strategy that most dieting gurus peddle on a frequent basis the "don't shop while hungry" and "always shop with a list" advice. But what other strategies could you put in place to up your game and ensure you become or stay a "loser" when shopping for your WLS regimen?

CONSIDER SHOPPING ONLINE

I'm not just talking about a weekly or monthly online shop for everything. This is something to consider for buying shelf-stable staples—oats, protein bars, canned tomatoes, dried fruit, canned beans, and much more. Many of the big shopping sites like Amazon, My Protein, Safeway, and Kroger have delivery programs that offer great value and ensure that you don't run out of those everyday items that make up the basis of your regimen. Shopping this way might even prevent you from making some junk food purchases you don't need.

PLAN YOUR MEALS IN ADVANCE

Why not sit down with a pad and pen and consider what you are going to eat for the next few days, then figure out the meals you wish to make or eat and build your grocery list around these decisions. For thriftiness, choose some meals with overlapping ingredients to prevent a pile-up of leftovers or half-used cans, and cut down on food waste. Before you leave for the market, check that list again by checking your cupboards, cabinets, fridge, and freezer, striking off anything that doubles up what you need.

STAY FOCUSED AND MINDFUL

I'm not saying that you have to plan your shopping like a military operation, but make this a determined "in and then out" maneuver. It's not the time to multitask and browse the shelves if you're determined not to be tricked into impulse buys, and don't be distracted by too many signs and requests to "sample" products. Idle browsing and chatting along with another shopper can also prove very distracting and can mean you come home without the one thing you really need.

BUY IN BULK

Only do this if a) they are items that you genuinely use regularly and can guarantee to use up before the use-by date, and b) the savings are really worth it and you won't be tempted to eat more of this item simply because it's there. I find a big-box store like Costco ideal for buying things like canned tuna, oatmeal, nuts, and frozen fish.

MAKE FRIENDS AT THE MEAT AND FISH COUNTERS

I find the assistants at these most helpful if you make friends with them. Most will weigh a very small quantity (that you can't get pre-packaged), butcher/gut/prepare meat to your exact requirements, and even for extra leanness, which saves you the chore later. Many also can advise on cooking times and methods as well as forewarn you of any special deals that day or coming up. For example, my local always has a special fish deal on Friday and a Saturday steak-night special that's worth considering.

TIMING CAN BE EVERYTHING

Some stores have now become so huge that it takes at least an hour to navigate them—so making small, frequent trips to a more local and smaller store may prove more time saving than you think. Otherwise, get to know your big store layout very well and go to just the aisles you need. Resist the urge to linger and stray into others when time is at a premium. I have found most of these aisles are on the periphery of the store, but there will always be one that is deep inside (store planners want you to stroll around)—locate it, bank it to your memory, and hope and pray they don't change it too often. Planning ahead like this and making a few more trips as opposed to massive occasional ones can help to ensure the food you purchase is super-fresh, and you'll cut down on or minimize food waste. Also, check out the produce at the back of a shelf. It's likely to have a longer expiration date than those positioned at the front.

CHECK OUT THE YELLOW STICKER FOODS

This is something I frequently do—delve through the discounted fresh food that needs to be sold that day and therefore can be marked down to a silly price. However, don't be tempted to buy everything there just because it's cheap. Fine, buy all those tomatoes if you plan to batch-make a sauce immediately, but don't if they are likely to be in the refrigerator staring at you at the end of the week. I often just select foods that I know can be frozen—that way I can choose the time-scale of use.

Getting Organized in the Kitchen

I agree with the saying "fail to plan, plan to fail" and can't emphasize enough that planning and getting organized in the kitchen is the best route to this new way of eating. The new regimen is so much easier to follow if your cupboard, refrigerator, and freezer are ready for it. Plus, check out your online supplier and set up a regular order of the things you often use, so that you don't run out or go too low at crucial times.

Likewise, if your kitchen has the gadgets you need to make food prep easy and light work then you have the head start on many. Bookmark recipes and meal ideas you like so that you can return to them quickly when time is at a premium.

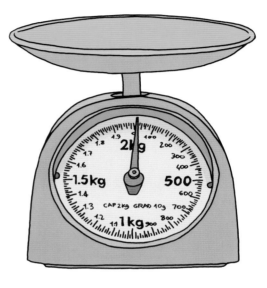

Basic Kitchen and Cooking Equipment

You won't need anything really special to get started beyond your regular kitchenware, but some extras do cut down on hassle and are probably worthy of the extra investment.

For essentials, you'll need kitchen scales, measuring cups, and measuring spoons. Ice cube trays and small freezer containers are very useful and also help to cut down on waste since you can freeze or store leftovers. I find a food processor or blender invaluable but you could consider a baby blender or single-portion type for coping with the Yellow (or soft food) stage.

Further down the line, I use, on a daily basis, nonstick cookware, which means I don't need to use lashings of oil to stop food from sticking during roasting or baking. Small ramekins and baking dishes have also proven to be an ally when cooking small solo-type meals both savory and sweet. Choose ones that can go in the freezer, microwave, and dishwasher for multi-use.

I also have purchased a small spray gun (the sort for misting plants) to mix water and oil for a simple but effective low-fat spray.

Specialized Kitchen and Cooking Equipment

There are so many gadgets out there. Your selection of indispensable ones will differ from mine since we might cook and enjoy very different foods and cuisines.

The items I find indispensable are an airfryer for cooking foods with minimal oil; a microwave for speed on almost every level—defrosting, reheating, and cooking; an electric ice cream maker—only probably justifiable if you like to make your own; and a slow-cooker, which means I can prepare in the morning (or the night before) what we will be eating some six to eight hours later.

You might add a rice cooker, herb chopper, electric bread-baking machine, or countless other gadgets—I have them all languishing in a cupboard but they may well be on your work surface and used every day.

LIGHTEN UP: COOKING TIPS

I still like to cook with a little butter and oil when the flavor is essential, but for a lot of dishes I use a low-fat spray. Using them can cut down appreciably on the fat and calorie content of a dish. There are a good few commercial varieties available and some with special seasonings like garlic and chile. I often prefer to make my own with water and oil (and herbs plus seasonings, sometimes) in a spray bottle which I keep in the refrigerator. Shake well before using to produce an emulsion.

Likewise, I sometimes use a low-fat spread or light butter instead of the real thing. I have enjoyed a good degree of success with them, and if they are mentioned in one of the recipes in this book, you can be assured they work.

It's tricky to give hard and fast rules about substitutions for fats and sugars, but for the former yogurt, banana, eggs, light cheese, quark, and applesauce can be useful, and I have used each and all of them to good effect (see the guidelines on pages 31–32). For sugar, I also use bananas, chopped dates, applesauce, low- or no-sugar syrups, granulated sweeteners and liquid ones.

For adding flavor when reducing fat and sugar (which are great flavor transporters), I use a multitude of herbs (fresh and dried), spices, rubs, sauces, mustards, purées, seasonings, and pastes. Low-fat and low-sugar cooking shouldn't be boring—this is a new regimen, not a *diet*. Many of these seasonings now come in ready-mixed form and are readily available from so many outlets.

Essential Portion Control

I've often felt like a cheerleader when I shout loud and proud about WLS, but the same can also be said about my feelings on portion size and control. I've always held it responsible (in a large part) for my obesity. I didn't eat a great deal of the "wrong" things prior to surgery (and I don't really hold with the notion of good or bad food) but I certainly ate too much of all kinds.

The key to my own weight loss I firmly lay at the door of my surgery (it gave me a tool I could work with), but portion control undoubtedly has been the foundation of my success with maintenance.

Portion Distortion and Portion Creep

You might be surprised to know that research shows that our portion sizes are 50 percent bigger than they were just twenty years ago! A scary statistic in its own right. Scarier when you think about the size of what could be an average plateful in 2040. But be honest—which one of these is you? Do you pile your plate high or go for modest helpings? Clear your plate clean afterwards or leave just a little to show you've had your fill? Chances are it's less to do with your actual hunger and more about your habits.

The fact is that most of us today are eating a great deal more than our parents or grandparents ever did. Not only are our average meal or snack servings now a whopping 50 percent larger than in the past, but the rise of processed foods—with all that added sugar and fat—means the food we eat now often packs a much higher caloric punch.

Of course, our modern tendency to pig out isn't helped by the fact that we're surrounded by temptation. Fast food on every corner, fries with everything, and cakes, cookies, and chocolate, all prominently on display—whether we are in the coffee shop, supermarket, or even the pharmacy.

What's more, the ready availability of junk food means unhealthy choices are much easier and cheaper to make than healthy ones. Enough to stretch our willpower to the breaking point.

A study at Exeter University using computer modeling found there seems to be no evolutionary mechanism to help us resist the lure of sweet, fatty, and unhealthy food, or prevent us from piling on the weight. That's because, in the past, being overweight did not pose a big threat to survival compared to the dangers of being underweight.

So our subconscious controls against becoming overweight are weak and easily overcome by the immediate rewards of tasty food—particularly in the winter when food in the natural world is scarce. Bad news for those New Year diets.

The more we overeat, the more our bodies expect, as our stomach stretches to accommodate these mega-portions of food. So if we don't watch it, bigger and bigger portions become the norm.

But the good news is that by reducing your portion size, you can shrink the size of your stomach to some degree—and train yourself to expect and want less food.

One way is to trick yourself into taking smaller portions is shown by a study confirming the benefits of smaller plate size. Over fifty studies have tested the effect of smaller plates on consumption. Researchers collated these studies and concluded that halving plate size does indeed lead to a 30 percent reduction in the average amount of food consumed.

Of course this isn't the whole answer—sadly, there's no such thing as weight loss on a plate per se! But if you're trying to shed the pounds (or avoid putting them on) it could be reason enough to splash out on a new set of dinner plates. And if you combine this with other techniques to develop healthier food habits, you'll be well on your way to managing your weight without resorting to fad diets that don't work.

These are some of the tactics that bariatric teams and bariatric dieticians recommend to patients after WLS. Most will recommend weighing food and checking individual portion sizes of specific foods using a small side plate or special bariatric portion plate or using any number of measuring aids to eye-check and validate what's being consumed.

MEASURING: TOOLS AND PRODUCTS THAT HELP

Most patients weigh and measure their foods assiduously for the first few months after surgery, and then, as they get further out from surgery, things begin to slip. It's somewhat tiresome to get the scales out, measure spoonfuls of ingredients or check the volume of food all the time. And herein lies the road to making mistakes, letting "portion creep" through the door, or enabling weight regain to be a reality.

Some people are very good at "eyeballing" a portion size, instead of measuring it, and there are some good visual reminders online that encourage us to think of a piece of protein as about the size of a pack of cards, or a cube of cheese about the size of a dice, but none are as accurate as getting out the scales, measuring spoons, and measuring cups.

I would always recommend that bariatric patients arm themselves with

- a set of *measuring spoons*
- a set of *scales*—mechanical with a dial or digital with an electronic reading
- a set of *measuring cups*—I like the ones that you can measure, cook, and serve in for absolute flexibility.

But real life can get in the way and sometimes it's good to use something that helps to get it "right enough." This is where the following really do earn their money:

- If you have a tendency to race your way through a meal, a set of *bariatric cutlery* may help to slow you down. These aren't kiddie cutlery—they simply have a smaller head, restricting how much you can load at a time. Children's cutlery isn't the same—it just has a smaller handle for tiny hands.
- A bariatric *portion plate* holds the ideal amount of food for the average post-op patient but also proportions it so that the correct quantities and ratios are applied for specific food groups. The most useful divide the plate for protein, vegetables, and starchy foods. I prefer to use a discreet one rather than an all-dancing cartoon one but there is one to suit all likes, pockets, and surgery types. I would advise that if you are an avid microwave cook, choose one that is non-melamine (which scorches in the microwave) if you wish to reheat a meal on the plate. Likewise, check that it can go in the dishwasher if that's your preferred mode of clearing up after a meal.

HOW TO USE A BARIATRIC PORTION PLATE

A bariatric portion plate, with indicators to ensure that foods eaten after surgery are in the correct proportions, is designed to help all weight loss surgery patients (regardless of procedure) eat the right ratio of food so that they achieve a healthy balanced diet post-op. It also gives a good idea if the portion size is too big and will hamper good weight loss or sustained maintenance. For those with a gastric band, it can also indicate if a meal is too large or too small and help with the decision of whether a band fill or de-fill is appropriate.

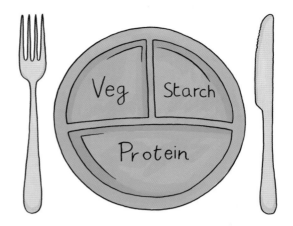

How to use

- Fill **half** of the plate with lean protein. This includes meat, fish, poultry, game, eggs, low-fat cheese, beans, lentils, nuts, and vegetarian options like soy protein, Quorn, and tofu.
- Fill **a quarter** of the plate with vegetables or salad.
- Fill **a quarter** of the plate with starchy foods like pasta, rice, potatoes, bread, couscous, and other grains. Ideally, choose whole wheat or whole grain varieties that have more fiber.

Eat only to the point of fullness

- Follow the 20:20:20 rule (see page 64).
- Try to eat at the table without distraction, "mindfully" eating your meal.

BARIATRIC BENTO BOX IDEAS

A bariatric bento box—smaller than usual (about half-size and divided for differing rations of food), will keep food safe and secure for travel and use away from home. There are many designs, colors, and sizes to suit all tastes and pockets. Those that come with a fork and have their own carrying bag that doubles as a placemat for "al desko" eating are helpful. An inner divider allows you to split up different foods and a sauce pot is ideal for dressings, sauces, or dips.

Some Bariatric Bento Box Lunch Ideas

Here are some easy bariatric bento box lunch ideas that keep items divided for freshness and crispness.

- A tuna, onion, and tomato salad with whole grain crackers
- A Greek salad with low-fat feta cheese, olives, and small whole grain roll
- A couple of shrimp and rice-paper rolls mixed with shredded vegetables and a low-fat and low-sugar dipping sauce
- A couple of spoonfuls of smoked fish pâté (made with low-fat cottage cheese) in the saucepot to serve with a small whole grain pita or cracker with salad
- A sliced flatbread with hummus, tabbouleh, or falafel
- A stir-fry of mixed vegetables with cubed tofu or meat and low-fat sauce (to be eaten hot or cold)
- A chickpea salad with ham or Quorn deli meat
- A lentil, beet, and cheese salad with separate low-fat dressing
- A savory low-fat muffin (e.g., ham, corn, and zucchini) with separate fruit salad

The 20:20:20 Rule

One of the best rules I was given and have been reminded of since surgery is the 20:20:20 rule. It simply means
- Aim (but don't exceed) to eat twenty mouthfuls of food for a meal over a twenty-minute period of time, chewing each mouthful twenty times, and putting your knife and fork down between each mouthful.

Other interpretations of this are
- Take a small volume of food onto your fork or teaspoon (no bigger than the size of your thumbnail.
- Chew the mouthful thoroughly (twenty times) before swallowing.
- Put your cutlery down, then count to twenty before putting the next mouthful in.
- Eat in this way for a period of twenty minutes. At this point, stop and walk away. Give yourself five to ten minutes and then consider whether you are still hungry; if not—stop eating. Discard any food that is left or save for another meal. Only go back to the meal if you genuinely still feel physically hungry—try three to four more mouthfuls eaten in the same way and then consider your hunger level again.

In others words
- Don't extend your meal to over twenty minutes unless genuinely hungry.
- Don't under-chew—make sure each mouthful you swallow has been well masticated to the consistency of applesauce.
- Don't race through your meal without "mindfully" eating it. Eat at a table or without distraction, whenever you can, too.

Reading and Deciphering a Food Label

Your WLS team will suggest that, post-op, you arm yourself with good nutritional food that complies with the less than 3 to 5 percent fat and sugar rule for healthy and bariatric-friendly meals as much as possible. That's fine if you follow recipes where the nutritional information is given, but what about ready-prepared dishes or those you cook yourself from scratch with packaged food components?

It helps to be able to read the back of the package to glean this information—but it's not exactly straightforward. Check out the handy guide that follows to help you decode the labels on your food. Learn how to spot the winners and swerve the binners.

INGREDIENTS

Yes, it's scary when most of the components of your favorite treats seem to begin with the letter "E," but the ingredients list should be your first port of call. Ingredients are listed in order of weight, so, if one of the top three is "sugar" or "hydrogenated vegetable oil," beware.

Added sugar can trigger blood sugar spikes and lead to weight gain—keep an eye out for all kinds of syrups, honey, nectar, molasses and anything ending in "-ose" (fructose, glucose, dextrose, maltose). Sugar is often added to foods labeled "low fat," "fat free," or "diet" to boost flavor. You should also watch out for artificial sweeteners such as aspartame, saccharin, and sucralose, which have been linked to weight gain and health problems.

Hydrogenated oils are vegetable oils which have been converted into "trans fats" as a result of chemical processing. Research (controlling for calorie consumption) has linked trans-fat intake to weight gain and abdominal fat storage, as well as to health conditions such as heart disease.

Seek out products made up of unprocessed, "real food" ingredients as much as possible. As a rule of thumb, the shorter the list, the better! Look for cereals, rice, pasta, bread, and wheat products made from oats, whole grains, or whole wheat flour (not simply "wheat flour"). However, beware of "natural flavorings." This can conceal hidden nasties like MSG (monosodium glutamate), which has been linked to obesity.

SERVING SIZE

That cheese-packed, carb-heavy frozen meal may "only" have 378 calories per serving . . . but take a closer look at the small print: the serving size is half a package. Oh. Food manufacturers' ideas of serving sizes (two squares of chocolate, for example) very often differ from ours (the entire bar). If you are going to eat the entire bar, and the entire bar contains ten squares, you'll need to multiply the values on the label by five (sorry, those are the rules).

CALORIE DENSITY

More calorie-dense foods are lower in calories, gram for gram, and tend to keep you feeling fuller for longer. If you are comparing two options, don't automatically pick the one with fewer calories per serving—see how they compare per 100 g, too.

FAT

Nutrition labels usually tell you what proportion of your daily reference intake of total fats and saturated fats a product provides. Fats provide essential nutrients, and a high-fat diet won't necessarily impede weight loss. In fact, the saturated fats in coconut oil have been linked to a reduction in belly fat. However, if the fat in your food is largely made up of hydrogenated oils (aka trans fat), you should be cautious of high values here.

SUGAR

Eating too much sugar may cause blood pressure spikes, which trigger cravings and encourage the body to store excess calories as fat, so it pays to watch your intake carefully. Nutritionists recommend you opt for breads and cereals containing no more than 10 g sugar per 100 g. Cereals containing dried fruit should contain no more than 20 g sugar per 100 g.

Limit added sugars (including honey) to 30 g per day, or no more than 5 percent of your daily calorie intake. However, you may safely consume some additional sugar in the form of fruit, according to most nutritionists (but not fruit juice, which should be limited to ⅔ cup/150 ml per day). Although an energy bar made from "raw" fruit and nuts may contain more sugar than a chocolate bar, for example, most nutritionists would advise you to pick the former—you should still try to see it as a treat, though!

SALT

A high-sodium diet can encourage water retention and bloating, so keeping your intake down could help you squeeze into those skinny jeans. A high-salt food contains more than 1.5 g salt per 100 g, while a low-salt food contains less than 0.3 g salt per 100 g.

FIBER

Fiber helps to fill you up, slow sugar release, and curb cravings. In one study, people who consumed an additional 14 g fiber at least two days a week lost an additional one pound over the course of a month. Experts recommend choosing breads, cereals, and snacks containing at least 3 to 5 g fiber per serving.

GET THE BALANCE RIGHT

A simple calculation could tell you how healthy your choice of meal or snack is, according to celebrity nutritionist Dr. Charles Passler. It all comes down to the balance between carbohydrates, fiber, and protein. Protein-rich foods reduce appetite, heighten our sense of satiety, boost metabolic rate, and curb carbohydrate-induced spikes in blood sugar. When choosing a meal or snack, you should aim for at least one part protein to two parts carbs (minus fiber).

You can use a simple formula to calculate the ratio using the values given in the "per 100 g" or "per serving" column. Simply subtract the fiber value from the total carbohydrate value, then divide the result by the protein value: *(Carbohydrates − Fiber) ÷ Protein*.

Coping Mechanisms

To Tell or Not to Tell

Many WLS patients deliberate over whether to tell friends, family, and the wider world about their surgery. Some are loud and proud and want to tell it the way it is from the start; others (myself included) just tell immediate family until they feel comfortable about their decision, and some choose to keep it to themselves.

There is no right or wrong action here—do what you think is best and what makes you feel most comfortable.

There's no doubt that you can miss out on support early on if you don't let others know, but the plus side is that you don't have to suffer a barrage of questions, unhelpful comments, or even total lack of support. It does, however, take some courage to deal with alone, even if you have a great deal of support from your bariatric team.

Some find their support outside their family, coworkers, and friends—in forums, support groups, and via buddy-sponsors. Many of these are private groups and will ensure privacy, but be aware that they do not guarantee it. If you wish to stay anonymous, opt for a username, and don't give any personal details away online, or post any identifiable pictures, however tempting it might be to show before and after ones!

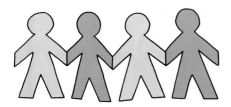

Support Groups, Forums, and Online Sites

There are countless WLS forums and support groups that you can join in person or from the comfort of your own home, online. Many groups are attached to hospitals or providers, some hospital-run, and others patient-led. Both are very useful, since they are often overseen by professionals or bariatric teams and advice is monitored accordingly. It also often means they are local to where the patient lives and offer face-to-face as well as online support near to home.

Others are run by charities, frequently have experts on hand, and are stringently moderated by admins who try as much as possible to give 24-hour support. They may be local, national, or international, and some are divided beyond the usual WLS assortment of surgery type, gender, pre-op/post-op/regain status, or interest (like recipes/cosmetic surgery/clothing swaps).

As with all groups of this kind, they are only as good as the people who run and moderate them. It's essential if you join one to never use their advice to override what your own team has told you. Some of the advice may not be right for you, not right for any WLS patient, and, at times, downright dangerous!

That said, there are many studies that show that attending a support group is advantageous and that patients who do engage often have more successful outcomes.

If there isn't a support group near you or online that meets your needs, then why not consider starting your own?

Setting Up Your Support System

It can be a tough call to stay motivated when it comes to sustained weight loss, maintenance, and fitness goals after WLS. Many coaches recommend that one of the best ways to stay motivated is to have a solid network of friends, family, and supporters to help you accomplish your goals. A support group can be wonderful if there's one that you can attend on a regular basis.

But what if there isn't a support group or it's held at an inconvenient time? What if your family lives miles away, friends aren't available 24–7, or your loved ones aren't as enthusiastic or as supportive as you'd like them to be?

With a little know-how, you can overcome these obstacles and put in place your own cheerleading support system for when the going gets tough. Here are a few ways to stay motivated on your own.

- Find yourself some *virtual friends:* Forums, message boards, and other online communities enable you to make friends with like-minded people regardless of where they live. Log on, listen, and if you feel like it, have a chat. Join and be "loud and proud," if that suits you, or join and listen-in for a while before asking questions or making a contribution.
- Set yourself a little *challenge:* Aim for something achievable that needs just a little extra push. Make it specific wherever possible. Perhaps one of your virtual buddies may join you in the challenge.
- Commit to a *weekly weigh-in* (but not more often): Even if it's just with a log-on weight-monitoring set up . . . it serves as a reminder of how far you have come. Alternatively, check in with a supportive member of your family or a friend once a week with a weigh-in update . . . it might be just what you need to help you stay on track.
- Set up a *reward system* for yourself: Throw a coin in a jar for every pound you lose or every exercise session completed, then use later for a healthy treat. Those coins can add up pretty quickly and will spur you on.
- Give yourself a *pep talk:* Just to reaffirm your goals from time to time; keep a journal that sets out your goals, struggles, setbacks, successes, and accomplishments; or take some photos or make a video diary that reminds you of your journey. It can be a great way to support yourself when there is no one else around to do so.
- Supporters don't just have to be people . . . enlist your *pet as your workout partner:* Think of your dog or horse, for example, as your daily motivator . . . they always need and rarely decline an exercise opportunity.
- Finally, *surround yourself with success:* Indulge yourself with feel-good stories of those who have succeeded in magazines, books, and TV or weight loss reality shows. Such stories can lift your spirits when motivation is flagging, and reading or watching how someone else has pushed through their limitations may be all you need to help you through some tricky times too. Steer clear of detractors who can quickly drain your resolve.

The Importance of Sleep

Healthy eating is important. Exercise is important. Food plans and regimens are important. But when it comes to balanced living and coping with all that life throws at us, too many of us forget an essential component: a good night's sleep!

Do you find it tricky to drift off into dreamland for a long, restful visit? These tips might help.

- *Go to bed earlier:* Sounds simple, doesn't it! But it isn't. And even if you go to bed early, many of us just lie there tossing and turning until we get to our "normal" bedtime. The trick is to take it slowly, patiently. Go to bed fifteen minutes earlier than normal every three days. Follow this routine religiously, and in less than two weeks you'll be enjoying an extra hour's sleep! Doing this will give your sleep cycle time to adapt, and will avoid the side effects (lying in bed awake) of a sudden change in sleep habits.
- *Turn off the screens:* It can't be stressed enough. Ideally, all screens—phones, computers, TV —should be off two hours before you turn in. For many, this isn't realistic, but try to give yourselves at least half an hour's break before you go to sleep. One easy rule to follow is to simply leave your phone in another room at night. (Buy an old-fashioned alarm clock if you need to.)
- *Avoid alcohol, sugar, and caffeine:* Avoid for at least two hours before you go to bed. If you are particularly sensitive to any of these stimulants, give them up entirely for a week or so, and track the improvement in your sleep.
- *Get outside during the day:* Do this as much as possible—sunlight regulates your body's production of melatonin which helps to regulate your sleep/wake cycle.
- *Make your room as dark as possible:* Do this when it's time to sleep. If this isn't an option, invest in the most comfortable eye-mask you can buy. Blocking out light really does help improve sleep.

If you find yourself lying in bed waiting for sleep to descend, here's a technique that really does work. It's called the *4-7-8 technique,* and requires two things— breathing and counting. Breathe in through your nose while you slowly count to four; hold the breath in for a slow count of seven; then exhale through your mouth for a count of eight. Do four cycles in all.

What Are the Signs of Real Hunger?

Once the "honeymoon period" is over after WLS (and sometimes before), when we mistakenly believe full-on, insatiable hunger returns, we have to ask ourselves, "Is this real physical hunger or something else at play?" I think the key to understanding this can be demonstrated in the checklist below.

Emotional or "head" hunger can be so easily confused with the physical kind. The key difference for me is that often emotional hunger comes on suddenly and is very food-specific (usually junk foods)—it might be different for you. Recognizing the difference between the two gives you the power to deal with it. Do you recognize any symptoms?

Real Hunger
- Comes on gradually
- Can wait for a bit
- Can be satisfied with a number of different options
- You feel satisfied and good afterward
- You stop eating when you're full

Emotional Hunger
- Comes on suddenly
- Requires immediate gratification
- You crave specific foods
- You can keep eating even on a full stomach
- You feel guilty, shameful, and powerless

Relationships After WLS

HELPING YOURSELF HELPS OTHERS

The weeks, months, and the first few years following weight loss surgery are filled with more changes than at most other times in life. Aside from the physical changes in your body, you'll often experience a number of changes in your primary relationships.

A percentage of people who have WLS follow the rules for maintaining a healthy weight after the initial weight loss period (the "honeymoon") and live life more fully than before WLS. It's very likely these people had healthy self-esteem before WLS. There are others, however, who struggle post-op as much as they did pre-op.

STRUGGLING WITH HEALTHY BEHAVIORS

After WLS, it is common for people to struggle with healthy behaviors. They struggle mightily with regain and often need to work through past issues and develop a healthier relationship with themselves in order to keep their weight off. They also need to work on healing their relationship with themselves so they can deal well with changes in other relationships after weight loss.

IMPROVING A RELATIONSHIP WITH YOURSELF

The most important thing you can do to improve the relationship with yourself is to work diligently on stopping negative self-talk. It's unlikely you will be able to do this alone—therapy with a licensed clinical psychologist or therapist is a good way to approach this.

RELATIONSHIPS WITH FAMILY MEMBERS

If a relationship was healthy going into the surgery, it will probably survive quite well after surgery. There are many very happy couples and families before and after WLS. In healthy family systems, people talk about the changes taking place and respect one another's emotional and physical changes. They talk about how they feel. They work together throughout the process of weight loss, adjusting to the changes together.

There are significantly more couples that were not working well together before one of the couple had WLS. These relationships are in jeopardy after surgery. The person who lost weight, particularly if they don't have a healthy self-esteem, will often do things in an effort to "make up for lost time." They may start dressing too young for their age, start drinking more and being too social, thereby disregarding their spouse and children's needs. Spouses of this type of WLS patient may get jealous or feel left out. In response, they may try to sabotage their partner's weight loss. The spouse who did not have surgery no longer feels needed or wanted by their partner. Many marriages that were unstable before WLS end in divorce after surgery.

CHANGING FRIENDSHIPS

Friendships also change many times after a person has lost a significant amount of weight. No longer do the "heavy or fat friends" of the WLS patient want to hang out with the person who lost weight. New friendships are started with others in the weight loss process or with people who had nothing to do with the person before they lost weight.

Those who have WLS and adjust to it well often experience an increase in self-esteem. As self-esteem improves, they start setting healthy boundaries with others and taking better care of themselves. In doing this, they may lose relationships with people who don't like the changes and make healthier relationships with people who respect them for setting boundaries.

Improved self-esteem often affects your relationships with other people in positive ways. Family and friends may be excited about the positive changes they see in how you treat yourself. In turn, they may want to spend more time around you and will likely treat you even better than they did before.

You can help your loved ones, if they feel threatened by the healthy changes in your life, by reassuring them, inviting them to join you in activities, and reminding them of their importance in your life. When they are more comfortable in their role within the relationship, they'll know better how to support you, and those relationships can actually start developing into deeper, more intimate ones. What a positive chain reaction—helping yourself often results in helping others! So do yourself a favor throughout your weight loss journey—improve your relationship with yourself and watch as other relationships in your life improve. *(Excerpts courtesy of Dr. Connie Stapleton)*

How to Help Your Loved One Before and After WLS

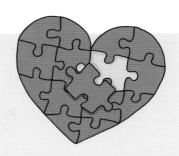

Pass this on to those who could support you . . .

If your loved one has decided to have WLS, it's extremely important that you give them all the support and encouragement that they need before surgery, afterward, and throughout their lifetime. They are much more likely to reach their weight loss milestones and achieve lasting success in maintaining their desired weight and a healthier lifestyle with the knowledge that you are fully behind them in their decision. Here's some advice on how to be the best support system you can be.

Educate yourself. You will need to know the facts about obesity and gain a good understanding about bariatric surgery, the options available to your loved one, their chosen surgery, and their reasons for making this life-changing decision. WLS is not an easy choice for your loved one and the path to success will undoubtedly be a roller coaster.

Make yourself aware of the limitations following bariatric surgery and reflect on how these could be made easier for your loved one. For example, your loved one will need to eat more slowly after surgery, so be patient and allow more time for meals.

Attend open evenings, support groups, and appointments with your loved one. Open evenings offer an excellent opportunity to learn about bariatric surgery and to ask questions in an informal setting. Often you'll have the chance to meet the surgeon and the team, too.

Support groups provide a comfortable way to learn more about bariatric surgery. Patients who have had WLS often attend, so you can hear first-hand their experiences, helping further your understanding of what your loved one can expect or may be going through. Having a forum where you can share information and experiences with a support network that offers mutual emotional support and understanding for both you and your loved one can be invaluable.

Attend aftercare appointments with your loved one. Actively participating in their weight loss journey shows how much you care while also providing you with helpful information that will allow you to have a greater understanding.

Keep the conversation going. Life after WLS can strain relationships as your partner changes physically as well as emotionally. A change in weight and health can bring uncertainty to a relationship as roles and responsibilities shift and evolve. Share your feelings and talk about how you can make changes together.

Offer emotional support. Your loved one may experience many different emotional states during their weight loss journey, including anxiety and depression. They may feel anxious about having surgery and keeping to a new lifestyle forever. After excessive weight loss they may feel extra confidence with their new body or feel vulnerable or afraid. They may become depressed when the reality of life after WLS does not match their hopes and expectations before surgery. They may miss social rituals such as eating out with friends. They may get tired of keeping to their diet and exercise program.

Your emotional support during these ups and downs will help your loved one get through them. Having someone to share their feelings with, who will listen and understand them while offering love and support will help lift them to higher ground so that they have the strength to continue.

Eliminate temptation. Many people must go on a special, very low-calorie diet before having weight loss surgery, to lose excess fat stored in the liver and enable the surgeon to carry out the operation. After weight loss surgery, it's essential that your loved one follows specific eating guidelines given to them by their bariatric surgeon or dietician.

You can help your loved one avoid temptation by keeping nutritious foods on hand and not bringing provisions into the house that your loved one shouldn't eat. Initially you might avoid pastimes that revolve around eating, such as holidays or meeting friends at a restaurant. Instead, you could suggest new challenges, such as walking a distance that your loved one was not able to do when they were obese, or inviting friends to your home for something other than food.

Diet together. It may prove valuable for you and your loved one to diet together. If you only eat foods that are inclusive of your loved one's strict diet, they will be more likely to stick to their new healthy-eating habits. They will appreciate your support, commitment, and dedication to helping them achieve their goals.

Encourage regular physical activity. Your loved one will need to make substantial changes to their lifestyle and, at times, they may not feel like doing the exercise required to ensure their weight loss continues. Often, WLS patients reach a plateau, and your support during this time will help them get over this hurdle. Become an active partner by participating in their exercise program. Offer to go for walks or bike rides with them. Often, sharing a new activity together is far more enjoyable and both of you will benefit from being more active.

Offer help. Talk to your loved one and find out if there is something they need or if they are struggling with a particular aspect of their new lifestyle. Together, you can decipher how to make it more manageable. For example, they may be struggling with their workload and new lifestyle balance and you may be able to help relieve them of some household chores to free up time for them to plan their diet and follow their exercise plan.

Focus on the positive and celebrate success. Always try to be positive and enthusiastic about your loved one's achievements, celebrating their successes along the way as they achieve weight loss milestones or embrace new lifestyle activities.

It can be difficult to change lifelong habits, and your loved one will have good days and bad days on their weight loss journey. Acknowledging the changes that your loved one has already made and offering encouragement and support will help keep them on track.

Regain and Plateaus

Can You Stretch Your Pouch?

Weight loss surgery patients and those considering WLS—particularly gastric-bypass surgery—are often concerned that they might "stretch" their pouch after undergoing the procedure. Bariatric patients who are several years out from their surgery also wonder whether they may have stretched their stomach pouch, since they no longer have the same feeling of fullness as they did in the first eighteen months after having WLS. Is it possible to stretch the stomach pouch created by a gastric bypass or gastric sleeve procedure? If so, what can be done to reverse the effects?

MANAGING YOUR POUCH

Your pouch will naturally stretch a little over time; however, it is generally unlikely that it will stretch all the way back to its original size. Although you may feel both physical symptoms as well as emotional remorse after an especially large meal, it is highly unlikely that you caused any permanent damage. That said, you are in control of your body and how you treat it. Here are some tips for managing your pouch to ensure you maintain a healthy weight for years to come:

- *Avoid overeating:* Before WLS, many patients wouldn't think twice about taking seconds, thirds . . . even fourths during a meal. After surgery, you may only eat a few bites because the 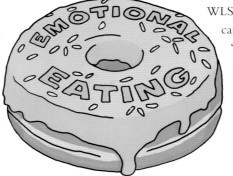 pouch makes you feel full with less food. In the first months after your procedure, note exactly how much you are eating to achieve that "full" feeling. Avoid helping yourself to seconds when your stomach is already at maximum capacity. Also, eat slowly to let that "full" feeling sink in. By measuring your food, taking your time during a meal, and being mindful of when you are full, you can avoid stretching your pouch.

- *Don't skip meals:* Skipping a meal will leave you hungry, and often you will find yourself grabbing the first snack available. Rarely are snacks grabbed on the go nutritious. Most people will reach for a chocolate bar instead of a banana at their local convenience store or supermarket checkout. Likewise, grazing on junk food, such as popcorn, cookies, and chips, is a sure-fire way to pack on a lot of calories without feeling full. You can avoid temptation by planning your meals, packing nutritious snacks when you're on the go, and making sure you stay on schedule with your eating.

- *Watch out for emotional eating:* Many people who struggle with obesity have a habit of emotional eating. They eat when they are bored, lonely, angry, happy, or stressed. In other words, they eat to manage their feelings. Although WLS can curb physical hunger, it can't do anything about your "head hunger" or appetite. Joining a support group and learning to recognize triggers and patterns can help you avoid emotional eating to ensure that you eat only when you are hungry and that you limit the food on your plate to the calories your body needs (not what your eyes crave).

- *Protect your stoma:* The stoma is the opening that gastric bypass patients have between the upper pouch and the intestine, which helps to regulate their food intake. If you don't chew your food thoroughly, or you wash large bits of food through the stoma with liquids, you can actually stretch this opening. If the stoma becomes enlarged, food will not stay in the pouch as long, and you will end up eating more because you never really feel full.

- *Avoid carbonated beverages:* Sodas and fizzy drinks are packed with sugar and high in calories, which can cause you to regain weight quickly and cause dumping syndrome, if you had a gastric bypass. Diet sodas have zero calories, but they still can cause you to regain weight. Numerous studies show that diet sodas trigger certain hormonal reactions that cause the body to store more fat. In addition, if you drink a carbonated beverage—even seltzer or soda water—while eating, it forces food through the stomach pouch faster. That means food does not stay in your pouch as long, and you lose the feeling of satiety, increasing the chances that you will eat more. Finally, the gas released from the carbonated beverage may cause the food forced through the pouch to enlarge your stoma, which would allow you to eat more at one sitting—defeating the purpose of the weight loss surgery. Stick with water, caffeine-free teas and coffee (in moderation), and other non-carbonated beverages for best results.

Remember that having WLS is not a get-out-of-jail free card, as far as your eating habits go. Long-term success requires long-term discipline.

Although your body might let you get away with a small cheat now and then, eating sweets, high-calorie foods, and carbonated beverages will have a detrimental effect on your weight and your waistline. Eventually, those bad decisions will catch up with you again.

Your best bet is to plan your meals in advance, avoid temptations, and connect with a weight loss surgery support group that can help you keep up all of your new healthy habits. If you find that you are eating larger and larger meals and that you are gaining significant weight over time, you may need to speak with your doctor about revision surgery.

Red Flags

Red flags are behaviors and habits that creep up on us post-surgery and often happen after the so-called WLS "honeymoon"—usually about nine months down the line.

The first sign is often a prolonged stall in weight loss (not to be confused with those weeks when you're still "doing everything right," and the scales don't register any loss, but you're still seeing a few non-scale victories). Or it may be a weight regain that is not going away, or is gradually getting worse. Maybe your appetite has returned and a few old destructive habits have resurfaced.

It's time to recognize these red flags and take immediate action. Here are some ways to do so.

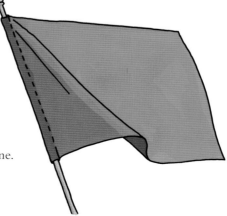

SNACKING AND GRAZING

In this scenario, a regular mealtime regimen has been substituted in part (or wholly by) a snacking and grazing one. So instead of three planned meals (and maybe two planned snacks) a "little and often" regimen has become more the norm. There are often several reasons for this—lack of planning, a mix-up of hunger signals, and tolerability issues of foods and their consistencies. Many patients find solid protein a challenge in the early days and find "slider" foods easier to tolerate. It's understandable to turn to something quick and easy (like easy-to-eat carb-based foods) for nutrition in a hurry or because you know it will "sit or settle well." But by adopting this regimen, you're setting yourself up for poor daily nutrition on all fronts—not enough protein, too many carbs, mixed fat messages, and often not enough fiber, vitamins, or minerals.

The Answer: Go back and reevaluate your regimen and make a conscious effort to plan and prepare meals with good solid protein as their basis. Keep grazer or "slider" foods and carbs well out of reach and plan a week's meals in advance to get back on track. It won't be easy, but it will be worth it.

DRINKING WITH MEALS

Many patients drift back to drinking with their meals—and not just water. The reasons for not drinking with meals have been outlined already but the temptation is still there. Likewise, it can also prove to be a gateway to cross-addiction-transfer, if it's alcohol that becomes a new habit.

The Answer: Go back to the 20:20:20 rule (see page 64) and don't drink 20 minutes before, 20 minutes after, or during a meal. Save the alcohol for special occasions, especially if you find it's becoming a regular habit. If you know you are struggling with this, it's better to be candid and seek help from your bariatric team.

AVOIDING THE SCALES

In the early days, many patients hop too frequently on the scales, and in the latter, too little. The urge to see the numbers decrease early on is a great motivator. When they don't move at all, or the numbers increase, patients tend to take one of two paths. Some see it as a signal to make change and reexamine their habits and regimen and others prefer the "ignorance is bliss" route.

The Answer: Don't become obsessed, but don't ignore the scales either. A once-a-week weigh-in is sufficient to tell you whether you're getting things right or not. Weigh on the same day, at the same time, in the same place, wearing the same clothes, for accuracy. Record this and use it as a tool to understand and adjust your regimen. It will quickly become clear what is working and what isn't. Write alongside your chart or journal what you did that week in terms of exercising, socializing, and cooking, to get some clues as to how to "tweak" your body to do the right thing. But remember, weight is only one aspect of your health—it isn't everything and the scales won't reflect that.

EMOTIONAL EATING

Head hunger, emotional eating, comfort eating, and mindless eating are all terms we are familiar with. During these times we don't reach out for the salad, fruit, or quinoa, do we? It may be that these were problems you thought were behind you after surgery only to find they rear their heads again later—a most unwelcome return guest. Whether it's carbs, cake, chocolate, chips, fries, candy, ice cream, pizza, or another trigger food, you may find they become "unwelcome friends" again.

The Answer: Acknowledge that they are a problem and then set about making some plans for how to deal with them when they raise their ugly heads. Diversionary tactics might work; having a little and limiting the damage is often another; or preparing a better alternative is a third strategy, which I follow. I don't say NO to pizza, cake, or ice cream (since it often makes me want them more) so I look for ways to make them more bariatric-friendly. You'll find many of these versions for trigger-type foods in the recipe section that follows. If you are suffering big-time with these, seek some professional help for binge-eating disorder from your bariatric team. Don't wait until it becomes so bad that you want to give up, isolate yourself, or undo all the progress you have made to date.

TRANSFER ADDICTIONS

Sadly, forums and anecdotal evidence from bariatric teams show that transfer addiction is alive and thriving within the bariatric community. These may be in the form of alcohol abuse, shopping addiction, decrease in sexual inhibition, fanatical exercising, gambling, or over-the-counter drug addiction. Usually, the WLS patient is aware of the problem and often prefers this addiction initially to the food addiction they hope they have kicked. In the case of alcohol, many will have a couple of glasses of wine instead of a meal; in the case of the exerciser, it's a means of controlling weight better than before, and often means food input can be increased without the weight gain; gamblers get their "hit" from a gambling high, rather than a food one; shopping can be thrilling when there is so much more to choose from; and, in the case of sexual encounters, many WLS patients will simply claim they are making up for lost time! All are highly dangerous in the long run. **The Answer:** Acknowledge that any excessive new behavior is equally as poor a choice as past eating behaviors, and make strides to reduce, control, or eliminate it. Most counselors will suggest the latter. First port of call should be your bariatric support team or MD for a referral to help with this. Don't delay.

Breaking Through a Plateau

So you have been losing weight successfully after WLS and then, all of a sudden, the numbers on the scale seem to stop moving. We're not talking about those "very early days" post-op and the small blips where the body is simply recalibrating, but longer term when you begin to doubt the loss will happen again. What next?

It's true that when we're actively trying to lose weight right out of surgery and feel almost invincible, we do all the right things—we eat well, hydrate excellently, exercise often, cut out snacks and grazing, don't drink half an hour either side of a meal—and we get great results. Then, the weight loss slows down, or we find that the number on the scales doesn't seem to be moving anymore. It might even go slightly north. Cue MASS PANIC! We look to exercise more, restrict all food groups, or indulge in one or two that we hope will have miraculous fat-shifting abilities.

So what do we mean by a "weight loss plateau?" The term refers to when your body no longer responds to your current diet and/or fitness regimen. Plateaus are often the result of the body developing a tolerance to the weight loss techniques that we are using, allowing the body to adjust and recognize the stresses caused and to slow down or even halt the effects and results. If you think you have hit one, there are five common signs to look for.

1. The scales aren't moving up or down.
2. You're doing the same things, but not achieving any new results.
3. You're bored with the food you're eating (or eating the same things monotonously) and fed-up with your workout or exercise schedule.
4. You find your exercise regimen easy or you're not breaking a sweat and feel like you haven't had a proper workout.

5. You lack motivation and aren't bothered about your meals or activity.

Sound familiar? Then here's what you can do . . .

THINGS TO TRY WHEN YOU HIT A PLATEAU

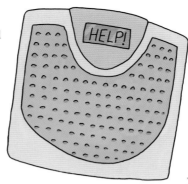

- *Monitor your weight loss off the scales:* Rather than focusing on weight loss, why not try checking your progress by something else more meaningful, such as a transformation photo with measurements recorded? You can take these every four or six weeks, and it will give you a better picture of what is going on without the stress and or trials and tribulations of getting on the scales daily or weekly. Wear the same clothes and you will start to see if they fit better, look baggy, or look different on a developing new shape.
- *Swap carbs and fats for protein:* Another option is to replace some calories eaten through carbs or fats with calories from protein. Upping the protein does seem to help most WLS patients. However, I can't stress enough the "some" part of this, as carbs are a necessity for a balanced diet. Protein helps with fat reduction, as it requires more energy to be broken down in the stomach, therefore increasing your metabolism. Protein also helps to suppress ghrelin, a hormone that stimulates appetite. It helps you feel fuller for longer. Try to spread your protein intake out throughout the day. Protein requirements will be unique to the individual and the surgery you have had. It's hard to calculate when malabsorption comes into the mix, but aim for 20 to 25 g minimum of protein at each meal (and, for duodenal switch patients, aim for much more—perhaps as much as 35 g). For example, 20 to 25 g can be found in a 4-ounce (115 g) chicken breast, or a protein shake.
- *Mix up your workouts and exercise regimen:* When it comes to exercising, muscles can become familiar with the same old thing, making your regular routine less effective. If you find that you are doing the same old, same old, it might be time to get out of your comfort zone and try something different—make your workout more challenging or introduce something new with a higher intensity.
- *Be super strict with your measuring, portion control, and snacking:* Don't let portion creep be the real winner here. Measure your food by weighing it, checking its volume, or using a bariatric portion plate, so that you get the quantities and proportions correct. If you're upping the protein (as in the second recommendation), make sure you use the full half-protein portion of the plate and "trespass" into the carbs area, too, until things get moving into loss again. And, while you may return to the one- to two-a-day healthy snacks (mainly to boost protein), give them a rest for now and just stick to your main meal regimen.

Pouch Tests: Fact vs. Myth

The "5-day pouch test," "3-day pouch reset," "2-week back on track regain reset regimen," and all other "reset" tests of varying duration promise to "reset" your stomach and help you lose more weight or counteract regain. The first is so popular it even has its own acronym in WLS forums—the 5DPT. So what's the deal? Is it too good to be true? Can it help? Do the experts endorse it?

The original test and subsequent variations are based on the observations of a gastric-bypasser who struggled with discouraging and disheartening regain after surgery. In an attempt to recreate that "tight newbie feeling of restriction," she developed the pouch test.

This test instructs you to "get back to basics" or, in other words, to return to the post-op liquid phase that is required immediately after surgery, then progress slowly from soft/puréed protein to firm protein, and finally to solid protein, over a five-day period. Following this, you are also supposed to feel a renewed sense of self.

Myths

The pouch test will not

- Shrink your stomach
- Reduce hunger and increase satiety
- "Reset" your body
- Cut your cravings for carbs and sweet/salty food

There are some good instructions within the test.

- *Always delay your fluids from your solid foods:* Stop drinking twenty minutes before your meals/snacks and wait at least twenty minutes after eating to start drinking again. Why? Drinking and eating at the same time "flushes" the food out of your stomach too quickly. This causes you to feel hungry soon after eating.
- *Take your time to eat:* Eating slowly and savoring your food without distractions increases satiety at mealtimes. Why? This gives your brain time to process that you are eating and lets you get the flavor fix you're looking for.
- *Ask yourself if liquid protein snacks (aka "slider foods") keep you full for long enough* (milk, yogurt, soft cheeses, cereal): While these foods are nutritious and provide good quality protein, they may not help you feel as full as you felt in the first few months after surgery. Why? These liquid foods spend less time in your stomach, which is why you feel hungry soon after eating.

- *Include a high-protein food at every meal and snack:* Why? High-protein foods help you keep fuller for longer.

According to most dieticians, these tests are just another diet in disguise. Anything that promises to "reset your system," "boost your weight loss," "cut cravings," "kickstart your metabolism," or "burn fat" is unfortunately wishful thinking.

There are no shortcuts to healthy eating and lasting weight loss. There is only you, your pouch (your smaller stomach), and knowing how to use it.

"How do I know if my pouch is still small?" Believe it or not, the majority of weight regain after WLS is NOT related to having stretched your stomach. The good news—weight regain is related to what you eat, the timing of your meals and snacks, and how you are eating. For example, if you feel comfortably full for two to three hours after eating the amount of food that fits on a side plate, which includes a combination of protein, a small amount of grains, and some vegetables, your pouch is most likely perfectly fine. So, you can reverse any regain, but not with a pouch test or reset regimen.

A bariatric WLS surgeon says: "The major reason for weight regain is the recurrence of unhealthy eating habits and/or lack of exercise. Maintaining weight loss requires a lifelong commitment to keeping up good habits and having support from your family, friends, and health-care team.

"I could not find any evidence or scientific papers about the five-day pouch test. Since it is not discussed in the whole of medical literature, even as a simple case report, I believe that there is no scientific basis for this reset diet. And simply thinking about how the gastric pouch and anastomosis works, it does not make logical sense to me how a five-day regimen of liquid and puréed food could possible shrink the gastric pouch. The original feeling of tightness immediately after surgery is probably because of inflammation, since the stomach was cut and stapled, and from the creation of anastomosis (suturing). This inflammation resolves after days/weeks during which the stomach is healing, and hence the original tightness feeling resolves with it."

—Dr. Simon Chow, bariatric surgeon, MD, MSc, FRCSC, FACS

(Information courtesy of Bariatric Surgery Nutrition)

Revisional Surgery: Why Some WLS Fails

It does appear that there has been an increase in revisions after bariatric surgery in recent years. It's still only a small percentage, but it's important that we look at failed outcomes and learn from them.

A recent European Obesity Summit indicated that pre-op selection for appropriate candidates and long-term post-op care, as well as new and continued lifestyle adherence by patients, are paramount indicators of good outcomes.

The main reasons for re-intervention are unsatisfactory weight loss or complications, and revisional surgery has been shown to be effective in providing good additional weight loss when performed to rectify these.

PREDICTIVE FACTORS

Several predictive factors have been identified as the causes of insufficient weight loss after surgery, including poor surgical technique (gastric pouch size, limb size), pre-operative weight loss, socioeconomic aspects, depression, behavioral factors, poor nutritional compliance, lack of physical activity, Type 2 Diabetes, and oral hypoglycemic agents.

POST-OP FACTORS

Post-operatively, patients must also understand the importance of adequate nutrition, increasing physical activity in their daily lifestyle (exercise regimen), stress management and setting realistic goals, and attending support groups, since many of these are reasons that surgery fails or does not bring the most successful results.

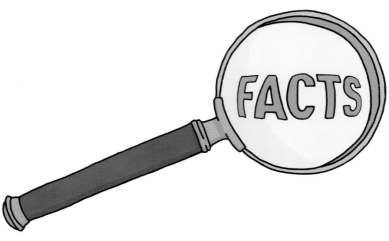

Four Tips to Stop Grazing

Studies show that grazing or mindless eating throughout the day is a common behavior of those who struggle with their weight and WLS patients are no exception to this. By grazing, little-by-little, snack-by-snack, you consume more calories than you need in a given day. This translates into unwanted pounds.

Constant grazing is a habit that can be broken. Often, our hurried lifestyles make it difficult to plan and prepare nutritious meals and snacks. We know what we should and shouldn't do; we know the dangers, but how do we break the grazing habit? Here are four simple but essential tips.

- Sit down once a week (when you are not hungry) to plan your meals and your snacks.
- Make a shopping list to get the things you need and if necessary, prepare a few meals in advance.
- Eat three meals each day and plan for two nutritious snacks each day, but otherwise avoid eating between meals.
- Make sure you have some low-calorie choices at the ready for unplanned hunger attacks. Consider low-calorie selections such as a piece of fruit, 100-calorie low-sugar yogurt, leftover steamed veggies, or a cup of bouillon or hot broth.

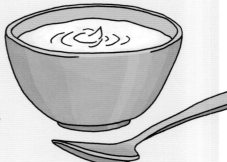

Back to Basics

I would undoubtedly say this is probably the most important information for post-op patients further down the line. We frequently say "get back on track" and "go back to basics." But what are they?

1. Eat three meals a day with a couple of optional small snacks that are high in protein, low in fat, and low in sugar. By that I mean under 3 percent fat and under 5 percent sugar—the only exclusions being foods with a high proportion of good fats, like avocados. Focus on solid protein that will give you satiety, rather than soft food that means you can eat more. So we're talking about cooked chicken, fish, meat, beans, low-fat cheese, and eggs. Other soft protein foods like yogurt, protein shakes, and cottage cheese, while being good sources of protein, should only feature once in a while since their texture is very soft and won't give you great restriction—so you'll get hungrier sooner.

2. Ideally, make your meal a minimum of 50 percent protein, 25 percent vegetables/salad and 25 percent starches/carbs, and eat in that order. Protein should always be eaten first and is your priority.

3. Use a bariatric portion plate or a small side plate to ensure your portion size is correct. Measure and weigh your food for portion control.

4. Do not drink twenty minutes before, twenty minutes after, or during your meal (see page 64). Hydrate well between meals so that you don't mistakenly experience what you think is hunger for thirst.

5. Do not demonize any food or food group—carbs are not bad—simply ensure you choose complex ones rather than simple junk food or heavily processed food. Likewise, good fats also have a vital part to play in a healthy post-surgery diet.

6. Eat a wide range of foods to ensure that you don't become bored with your regimen, and nature will ensure that it has the virtues of healthy nutrients, variety, and low cost, if eaten seasonally.

7. Follow the 20:20:20 rule regarding eating over a twenty-minute period of time (see page 64). If you have a tendency to eat too fast or take too large a mouthful then consider using portion-controlled cutlery.

8. Take your multivitamins, calcium, and any other prescribed supplements daily—it's vital for good ongoing health.

9. Not all foods will suit and you may have a low tolerability to some—but keep trying them and cook them in different ways. Don't fall into the trap of grazing on "slider foods" (see page 46) that are easy to eat but offer little nutritional value, and will hamper your loss and may lead to regain.

10. Incorporate some exercise into your daily activity as soon as you are able to do so. Look for something you enjoy and will do—no point joining a gym if you won't go or taking up swimming if you don't like to get your hair wet. The simplest, walking, is a good one since it requires little specialized equipment. There are, however, classes and workouts for all levels of ability and disability.

11. Surgery will fix the "pouch" but it doesn't fix the head and after WLS many patients still have problems with emotional eating. This is by no means rare and there is help around—just ask!

12. Likewise, some patients do experience problems with addiction transfer and help should always be sought if this starts to become a problem in your post-surgery life.

13. No doubt some will be worrying that they have stretched their pouch, and will ask about revision surgery. It's rare for this to happen, and for most, if you're still alive and kicking, then you can face your regain, own

it, and move on again with this "back to basics" set up. I know countless patients who have lost their regain by sensibly following the regimen they were initially given, getting back in the saddle with these basics, and losing weight again—even years after surgery. Revision patients will still have to go back to these basics and relearn what is successful and what is not.

14. Seriously consider joining a support group—at your hospital or a responsible online community with a great admin team to oversee postings and advice.

15. Keep experimenting with food, check out advice, and make your post-op life better than your pre-op one.

16. Eat mindfully by sitting at a table, using a knife and fork or spoon, rather than while mindlessly watching TV. Savor each and every mouthful and chew well, then chew some more . . .

17. Plan your meals and shop when you're not hungry or likely to be tempted with poor choice foods. Plan your meals away from home with care. Check out restaurant menus and workplace cafeteria options ahead of time, or take along a packed lunch box meal.

18. Plan and record your food intake (as well as exercise). A journal will help with this and is good for monitoring when things go right as well as wrong.

19. This is a regimen for life so make your food work for you—look for bariatric-friendly versions of your favorite meals—there are many in this book to make a good start.

Coping with Vacations, Eating Out, and Meetings

Ten Ways to Stay Healthy and on Track on Vacation

Leaving behind the era of guilt-inducing fly-and-flop vacations, more of us are now adopting the view that taking time off for your vacation shouldn't have to mean taking time off from your healthy lifestyle and throwing away months of hard work at the gym on one gluttonous getaway. This is especially true for those who have had WLS—who know how easy it is to veer away from the bariatric routine and so easily get off-track. You also don't want to sabotage your efforts with the wonderful tool that WLS brings, for it is just that, a "tool," and we still have to be vigilant about our choices, even on vacation.

Here are some tips that might help you to focus on health, exercise, and workouts during your time away.

- *Travel healthy:* Give yourself the best start and arrive at your destination in peak condition by traveling healthy. Being confined to the cramped conditions and recirculated air of an airplane can have a detrimental effect on your body and immune system. Swap boozy beverages for water to stay hydrated and keep your circulation flowing with some simple yoga stretches.

- *Be workout-wear prepared:* It may seem obvious, but this is a golden rule, so you can't use the fact that you don't have your sneakers or something suitable to wear as an excuse not to exercise. If suitcase space is an issue, pack a couple of workout wear options made of lightweight, breathable materials that can cope with the heat and can be easily hand-washed for re-wear during your trip.

- *Active exploration:* Adventure beyond the hotel pool and explore your new surroundings while giving a healthy boost to your fitness. Whether you'd rather take in the sights on a leisurely jog or go the distance on a bike ride, ask the concierge for the most picturesque route and discover the beautiful scenery while upping your heart rate.

- *Swim for success:* A full body workout and great cardiovascular exercise, swimming is a refreshing way to keep active while staying cool, and is full of health benefits, from muscle toning to reducing stress. Raise the pace and get your heart pumping by fitting in a few swift lengths in the pool or ocean before breakfast when there are fewer people around.

- *Catch up on sleep:* Constantly trying to shake the feeling of being overtired? Holidays are an important time to catch up on lost sleep and allow our bodies time to recover and recharge. Keep in mind that in hot conditions, sleep may be disrupted while your body adjusts to the new climate, so avoid the temptation to stay up late every night of your vacation.

- *Eat the right diet for the right vacation:* When leaving behind your usual routine, think about fueling your body with the right nutrition for your trip and not just reverting to the vacation mindset of overindulgence. If you're going on a multi-activity vacation, you'll need a diet of slow-energy-releasing carbohydrates in the correct bariatric proportions to keep up your strength. If you're relaxing on a spa break, watch your portion sizes and swap foods that are high in obvious sugar and fat for more fresh fruit and vegetables. If you're unsure about any buffet-style food, ask for details or steer clear.
- *Get some vitamin D:* The vitamin D we get from sunlight allows us to absorb the calcium and phosphate that makes our bones healthy and boosts our immune system. Outside of the peak hours of 11:00 AM to 3:00 PM, when the sun is at its hottest, spend fifteen minutes a day outdoors without sunscreen, to get your daily dose of vitamin D.
- *Use nature as your gym:* Make the most of your natural surroundings and embrace the opportunity to get out of the gym and back to nature. Add some resistance to your run by running a sandy beach, use the jungle as your own jungle gym, or take your workouts to the water with surfing or paddleboard yoga and discover muscles you didn't even know you had.
- *Cool down:* If you're exercising in hot conditions, your body's core temperature will be elevated. In order to recover effectively from a workout in the heat, bringing your core temperature down is a priority and will help to lessen muscle fatigue. Reducing your core temperature can also help you to recover sooner from the mental fatigue of a session.
- *Make day-to-day changes:* Health and fitness is a lifestyle and should be a part of your daily practice no matter where you are in the world. Make small daily changes on vacation, from taking the stairs rather than the elevator, to swapping an afternoon at the bar for a game of tennis or golf, and reap the rewards when you transition to your daily life back at home.

Some Travel Food Solutions for Road, Train, Air, and Sea

During summer and winter vacation time, there can be many temptations that make it harder to stick to the bariatric diet. One way to stay on track is to prepare for your trip with healthy snacks. Here are some bariatric-friendly snacks that can be pre-packed or purchased at the airport or gas station during your travels.

100-Calorie Nut Packs: Nuts are loaded with healthy fats, protein, and fiber to keep you fuller for longer. Though nuts are good for us, they are a high-calorie food. Purchase pre-portioned packs or portion out nuts in small bags to prevent overeating.

Homemade Trail Mix: Making your own trail mix helps to control the sugar content, which may be higher in pre-packaged trail mixes. Try mixing your favorite nuts and seeds with a few dark chocolate morsels or dried fruit for a sweet mix. You can also try adding spices such as cinnamon, nutmeg, or even cayenne pepper to mix up the flavor of your trail mix.

Beef or Turkey Jerky: Though beef jerky and turkey jerky are loaded with protein, they also contain a lot of salt to help preserve the meat. Stick to small portions of jerky, drink plenty of water, and eat fresh fruits and vegetables to balance out the sodium content.

High-Protein Chips: If you really need something crunchy to munch on during your trip there are a few brands of bariatric-friendly chips to try. The best places to purchase these high-protein, low-carbohydrate chips are online or at your local vitamin and supplement shop. Try searching "bariatric chips" on the internet to find the brand and flavor that suits you best! Or make your own (see Snack Attack Microwave Chips, page 229).

Individual Peanut Butter Packets with Whole Wheat Crackers: Individual peanut butter or other nut butter packets are an easy way to stick to proper portion sizes. Pair with whole wheat crackers for a quick and easy snack.

Other Great Snacks: Packing a cooler for your trip? Here are some high-protein snacks that are best refrigerated.
- Protein shakes
- Fresh fruit
- Cheese sticks
- Low-fat cheese and crackers
- Low-fat yogurt

Remember, going on vacation does not mean giving up on your diet. Packing ahead of time ensures that you are prepared for whatever eating challenges arise. Continue to choose healthy options wherever you go and enjoy your vacation!

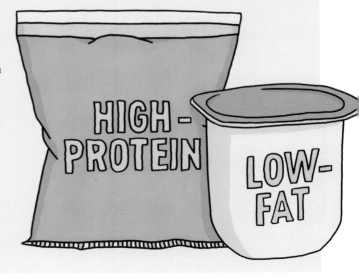

Best Bets at a Buffet

Roadside buffets, cafés, and work cafeterias all present many dilemmas for the WLS patient—not only because of the food choice but also because you don't know how the food has been cooked. It's often best to play safe and be very unadventurous—even the reliable salad bar can be a minefield of errors. Here are some suggestions.

Choose wisely at the salad bar. Making the right choices at a salad bar can be a good way to maintain your healthy eating plan. Help yourself to filling, non-starchy vegetables like broccoli and cauliflower and go easy on the cheese and salad dressing (olive oil and vinegar is a good choice; just remember that 2 tablespoons is the right amount to use for dressing salads). Top salads with good quality protein like chicken, deli meats, beans, or flaked fish.

Go for healthy soups. Soups are a healthy and filling cafeteria or buffet option when they are made without cream and with a variety of nutritious ingredients, such as vegetables, lean meats, poultry, or seafood, beans and other legumes, and/or whole grains like quinoa and barley. Try a black bean soup, or a soup made with broccoli or cauliflower in a beef, chicken, or vegetable broth base. Chilled tomato- or cucumber-based soups, like gazpacho, are also a good option in warmer months.

Check out the "made to order" stations. Some cafeterias and buffets offer individual stations that allow you to select the ingredients for your own omelet, pasta dish, or stir-fry. If you want an omelet, your best bet is to fill it with vegetables like peppers, tomatoes, spinach, and broccoli. If you want cheese, make sure it's reduced-fat or "mature" so you need less to get a great taste. For stir-fries, go for grilled/broiled chicken breast, shrimp, tofu, bok choy, broccoli, green beans, peppers, and/or mushrooms and make sure the "frying" oil is used sparingly, if you can. If you're ordering pasta, stick to a small half-cup serving of whole wheat pasta and choose a marinara, pesto, olive oil and garlic, or white wine-based sauce with just enough to coat the pasta but not drown or drench it. Avoid stations serving white pasta, burgers and fries, breaded chicken, and pepperoni pizza.

Postpone or forego dessert. Many of the desserts in cafeterias and buffets are healthy-eating regimen-busters and can be dumping ground territory with their high fat and high sugar offerings. Wait until the end of your meal to select a sugar-free Jello cup or fruit salad or limit yourself to just a bite or two of a decadent dessert (why not share with a friend?). Better yet, avoid temptation and wait until you get home to have a bariatric-friendly dessert you've prepared yourself.

Ask for it if you don't see it. If you'd like your chicken breast without the creamy sauce or you wish there were broccoli on the salad bar, speak up! Often food managers can accommodate special orders and meet your requests. Likewise, if you want your sauce, dressing, or topping on the side so that you can add the right amount yourself, just ask.

How to Eat Out, and In Other People's Homes, After WLS

I enjoy going out to eat. Whether it's eating in a restaurant or at a friend's house, you can count me in. It's one of my favorite things to do with my family and friends. Restaurants make the experience easy since it's possible to choose off a menu, but eating at someone's house can be more problematic. With some simple strategies, preparation, and a bit of discipline, dinner out or at a friend's house can be an enjoyable and a diet- or WLS-friendly experience! Here are a few ideas on how to strike a balance.

- *Pick and choose:* When dinner is served, focus on protein, then veggie dishes, salads, and finally carbs. Politely pass on anything that's smothered in sauces, cream, or mayo. If you do decide to indulge in a rich main course or a dessert, stick with a single, sensible, and ideally measured portion if you can.
- *Bring your own dish:* If dinner is buffet or potluck-style, bring nutritious, diet- or WLS-friendly options such as a healthy protein or vegetable dish, crudités platter, or fruit salad. This way you'll have something "safe" to eat, and you'll be sharing the gift of health!

- *Watch your hands:* If there are munchies within your reach, be sure to have only a single small portion instead of repeatedly reaching for a bowl or grazing before the main event. Hold a glass of water or carry a clutch bag with one hand so it's harder to pig out.
- *Be careful with the cocktails:* Alcoholic drinks can be loaded with calories and sugar and lower your inhibitions so you eat more. Some are so sugar-laden you may run the risk of "dumping" (see page 40). Have a glass of wine or a white wine spritzer—half wine, half seltzer (shaken very well to keep the fizz down)—instead of a sugary cocktail.
- *Inform the hosts:* Sometimes we feel pressured to eat because we think friends will be insulted if we don't. Before the dinner party, tell your host not to feel bad when you don't try everything or ask for seconds. Let her know that you're trying to cut down, have a regimen to follow, and not all the yummy dishes are on your menu.
- *Or keep quiet:* Whether they do it consciously or not, some friends and relatives sabotage our best intentions to live a healthy life. And pressure from family and friends can actually work against you staying motivated and slim. If your host is that type, don't fill her in on your way of life. Instead, think of a few things you can say, such as that you had a big or late lunch, when she pushes a fattening or unsuitable food on you.

You can also politely take a serving and leave it on your plate. Just because it's there doesn't mean you have to eat it.

- *Enjoy the company:* The reason we gather with friends is to share their company and conversation, and, in our go-go-go world, spending time with loved ones is rare. Instead of focusing on food, pay extra attention to those around you. You won't overindulge, and you'll connect with others in a meaningful way.

- *Look before you eat:* If the dinner is buffet, survey the whole spread before you choose what you'll eat. Use a small plate so you don't overdo it.

- *Offer your assistance:* Helping a friend prepare, serve, and do other things at the dinner may keep you too busy to munch mindlessly. Plus, you'll get a bit of exercise getting up and down or going back and forth to the kitchen.

- *Don't go hungry:* Some people starve themselves all day so they can eat what they want at a dinner, party, or special occasion. The problem? You'll be so hungry when you arrive at your friends' place, you're likely to make poor food choices and leave with an aching tummy and loads of regret. Stick with healthy meals during the day and, if you're pre-op, eat a filling snack right before you go to the party.

- *Stay focused on your goals:* When others around us are pigging out, it's all too easy to follow their lead. A study done at Vanderbilt University found that, on average, women took in 696 calories when they ate with others compared with 476 when they dined alone. But that doesn't mean you should shun social meals. Just remember that your goals are different from your friend's. Just because a girlfriend is reaching for seconds, doesn't mean that you have to. What one WLS patient can eat may also not be what another can, depending upon surgery type, time out from surgery, constraints of their bariatric team, and tolerances.

- *Think before you eat:* Before diving into that decadent dessert, imagine how you'll feel if you step on the scale and it's gone up or hasn't budged, or if your clothes are snug. Often the momentary pleasure is not worth the guilt you'll feel later. That said, if you do, draw a line under it and start again tomorrow with more resolve.

Survival Tips for Office Meetings with Food

I know of so many WLS patients who cope well until the office vending machine or obligatory cookie plate makes an appearance. What to do?

Meetings are the bane of corporate life. They are inevitable and sometimes a waste of time, but we're stuck with them. And for WLS patients, a major problem is the food and drinks often laid out for participants.

These seemingly harmless snacks encourage grazing and add needless calories to your daily tally. Often, they are low in nutritional value, like soft drinks, potato chips, cookies, or other sweets. Some offices offer water and fruit as well, but it's hard to compete with a plate of chocolate chip cookies!

Here are four survival tips.

1. Ask your company's HR department to provide healthy snacks for meetings—nuts, fruits, and unsweetened beverages.
2. Bring your own snack and water bottle to the meeting.
3. Sit as far as possible from the food.
4. Go to fewer meetings if you can—ask yourself, "Is this one essential?" Bow out if you decide it isn't and can do so.

Exercise

When and How Do I Start?

Exercise is advised both pre-op and post-op. Pre-op, you will be encouraged to up your activity and exercise levels so that the transition later is more manageable. It can also make surgery easier and safer (by decreasing your body fat). Afterward, when advised to do so, you can pick up on activity and exercise to increase your chances of success with weight loss but also movement and well-being.

Building activity into your life after WLS is considered one of the cornerstones of success and matters a good deal when it comes to maintenance further down the line.

If you've never exercised before, or only infrequently, you will need to start out slowly and safely.

- *Start before surgery* for all the reasons mentioned above.
- *Begin with simple walking:* This is a great way to start and can gradually be increased as time progresses. It's low-cost, almost everyone can do it, and it doesn't require too much in terms of special equipment. Most teams say that this can start at about six weeks post-op.
- *Discuss exercise with your bariatric team:* They will advise when you can start, when to move onto something more strenuous, and when to hold back if there are risks.

- *Do five to fifteen minutes of cardio before strength training:* Warm up your body first with a short cardio workout before moving onto strength training that will help build muscle mass.
- *Start off with one to two sets of six to fifteen repetitions:* Start small and build up, so you're not putting your body under undue stress.
- *Don't overdo the weights:* Tempting as it might be to push yourself, just do enough to feel resistance.
- *Keep an exercise log or journal:* This will help you monitor your progress, highlight your successes, and keep you on track.

What Is the Best Exercise?

In a nutshell, it's the one you enjoy and will do. Don't make swimming your main choice if you don't like getting your hair wet; forget the gym if you won't go because it's too far away; and put cycling on the back burner if you haven't learned to ride a bike. Consider instead any number of activities from aqua-aerobics to Zumba and everything in between. Some can be organized exercise, while others might be housework or garden- or shopping-related. Look at the free and low-cost options that are out there—a quick internet browse will tell you of many free park runs, low-cost boot camps, and leisure and swimming deals. Make time for this important tool in your weight loss armory. Set your alarm for twenty minutes earlier and just do it!

The following are some small ideas that will bring big differences:

- Try walking or cycling rather than using the car.
- Walk your dog or your neighbor's dog each day, and for a little longer than expected.
- Get off the bus a stop earlier and walk the rest of the way to your destination.
- Use the stairs instead of the elevator or escalator.
- View housework, shopping, and gardening as a workout rather than necessary chore.
- Strap on a pedometer or use an app to measure your steps or energy expenditure over a day and use it as a motivational aid.
- Consider some exercises you can do at your desk if you're in an office environment, or look at office exercise classes.

Exercise Goals

For the best results and ideal outcomes, experts suggest the following:

- Have a focus.
- Set yourself some manageable goals.
- Make exercise a top priority.
- Have a support or exercise buddy for when you don't feel like doing anything or enthusiasm wanes.
- Adopt a "can-do" attitude.
- Keep things in balance and remember there is no winner.
- Be accountable.
- Choose activities you enjoy and won't give up on easily.
- Be consistent.

Five Ways to Exercise at Home

It can be hard to find the time and space to exercise, especially if you find it hard to get out of the house or feel shy about working out in public places. The trick is to find something you can easily fit into your daily life so that it becomes routine. The gym may not be your thing, but here are five exercises that you can rely upon to get in shape and are easy to do at home. Once you have been given the go-ahead with your bariatric team to exercise, why not give them a go?

These exercises can help you tone up and burn calories. They will also help you feel and look fitter, as well as stronger, balanced, and more energetic. Ten minutes is a good starting point, but if that's difficult, try just one exercise. You can increase the length of the routine as you get fitter. The bonus is that you don't need any specific exercise equipment to do them either.

And to keep you motivated: Plenty of studies show that playing the right sort of music can boost your workout. Try an ultimate workout playlist as you do your workout.

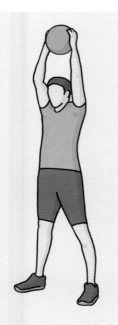

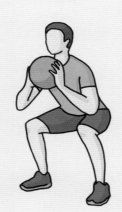

SQUAT

Target areas: abdominals, hips, thighs
Equipment: Ball or hand weights (optional)

Stand with feet apart. Place a ball between your hands. Gently draw in abdominals and slowly squat down, bringing knees to an 80 degree bend. Then slowly stand. Repeat three sets of ten.

To make it harder: Hold weights in your hands—a can from the cupboard weighing approximately 1 pound (500 g) can act as a small weight. You can increase the weight you carry as you get fitter, or use a backpack on your back with books in it to increase resistance. Lift one leg a little off the ground, and try to do this on one leg only.

STATIONARY LUNGE

Target areas: abdominals, hips, thighs
Equipment: hand weights or kitchen cans (optional)

Step one foot in front of the other: front foot flat on the ground, back foot up on your toe. Gently bend knees, then straighten. Bend your knee up to 90 degrees, but no further. The front knee should not go past the front toe: keep it centered over your foot.

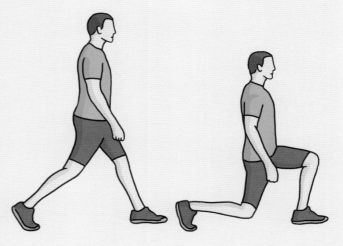

Repeat for thirty seconds with one leg leading, then for thirty seconds with the opposite leg leading. Do this cycle as many times as you wish.

To make it harder: Hold weights in your hands. Do the exercise slowly, pushing through the front heel more. This makes hip muscles work harder. Try a "stepping lunge." Walk lunge forward, lunging with one leg, then moving straight into a lunge with the opposite leg. Move forward for thirty seconds, then turn around and return to the start position. Now repeat.

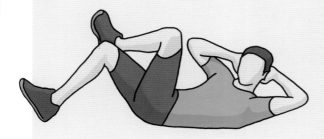

DIAGONAL SIT-UPS

Target areas: abdominals, trunk

Equipment: none

Lie on your back, knees bent, with one leg crossed over the other. Place hands on the side of your head. Lift the upper body and turn body to one side, then return to the midline. It is important to keep the neck straight and avoid bending the head forward. This targets the waist, giving you definition through the midriff. Start with between ten and twenty repetitions each side.

To make it harder: Do the exercise slowly. Keep your upper body off the ground in between sit-ups.

PLANK

Target areas: abdominals, trunk

Equipment: none

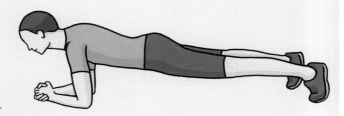

Place the elbows on the ground, directly underneath the shoulders. Rise up onto your toes so that your body stays straight and parallel to the ground. If you find it too difficult to raise yourself on your toes, try supporting yourself on bent knees instead. Gently draw in the abdominals. Clasp your hands together. Hold this position for ten seconds. Repeat five times.

To make it harder: Increase the length of time you hold the plank—up to thirty seconds is good, but make sure you don't lose your form. Keep your hands clasped and lift them off the ground, coming up higher on your elbows.

ARM TONING

Target areas: shoulders, arms, postural muscles

Equipment: hand weights or kitchen cans

Stand tall. Place small weights in your hand, 1 pound (500 g) to start with. You can use tins from the cupboard if you don't have weights. Place elbows at 90 degrees and bend the arm up, then take it back to 90 degrees. Repeat three sets of ten for each arm. Keep an upright posture to get the most out of this exercise.

To make it harder: Extend your arms straight out in front of you, level with your shoulders, palms with weights facing up. Bend your elbows fully, then return to the starting position. Increase weight or number of repetitions.

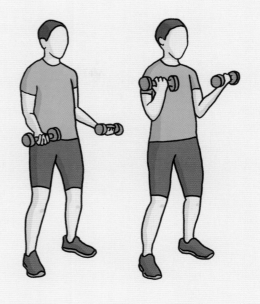

PHEW, YOU'RE DONE . . .

Congratulations, you've given your body a home workout. These exercises can help you feel stronger and are a good base from which to build toward other fitness goals. Alongside eating well and leading a healthy lifestyle, they help you burn calories and achieve a healthy weight. Do this routine at least two or three times a week and you'll soon see and feel the difference—not just in your fitness levels, but in terms of looking more toned and in shape.

Five Ways to Stay Active in the Winter: A Cold Weather Regimen

When it's grey and gloomy outside, and the days are short, it can be hard to motivate yourself to get up and do exercise. In the lead up to Christmas, we are also more likely to eat more of the less healthy options. Between mulled wine, heavy food, and lack of exposure to sunlight, it's easy to gain weight and feel sluggish. The same can be said for after Christmas before the longer days of spring arrive. Here are five top tips for staying active over the winter months.

Brave the Weather: It's easy to be put off, but going outside is all in the preparation and attitude. Wrap up warmly, wear decent footwear, and once you're out there, you might even enjoy it! Cold conditions give a boost to the conversion of white fat cells to brown, which burn energy to keep us warm. Outdoor exercise increases exposure to daylight and vitamin D, helping to increase endorphins, and improving both your mood and bone strength.

Exercise Indoors. If the weather really is appalling, try an exercise video or repeatedly going up and down the stairs.

Gyms often have tempting trials or short-term deals, and many gyms are reasonably priced. The price of exercising indoors is an investment in your long term health that's worth paying.

Ditch the Excuses. Modern life is busy, with work and family often taking priority. It's easy to think you have too many other things to do and that it's selfish to take time out. But studies show we are more efficient at work if we make time for exercise, and the "head space" helps with thinking and prioritizing. Exercise makes you healthier and happier, improves concentration, and increases energy levels.

Exercise with Others. It can be hard to get going on your own. Going for a walk with a partner, friend, or family makes it more pleasant, and meeting up with someone helps make sure you stay committed. It's a great way to make new acquaintances and catch up with old ones.

Set Goals and Monitor Yourself. You are more likely to be successful in maintaining weight or losing a few pounds if you know what your goals are and you record what you do. You can do this manually, or use technology to help. Activity can be monitored by a wearable device to record how many steps you take, how much ground you cover, and even how much sleep you have. Most health studies recommend 10,000 steps a day. You might be surprised by how little or how much you do, and how much small things like using the stairs, a ten-minute walk at lunchtime, or walking the kids to school can make. You can also use apps to map your activity and distance covered in a walk or run. Looking at your progress can be really motivating.

Practical Tips
- Choose to do an activity that is realistic and that you enjoy so you can keep it up.
- Wear appropriate clothing and stay well hydrated.
- Don't exercise if you feel unwell.
- Don't be too hard on yourself—it's winter but also party season! If you have a little too much to eat and drink, have less the next day and work it off.

On and Off the Scale

Weighing Yourself

Until I had WLS I used to be a veteran weighing-in robot—I would jump on the scale every time I went to the bathroom, and sometimes make special scheduled visits to check on progress. My whole day would be dictated by them! When that dial went down, my spirits soared, and when it moved up, my well-being shrank.

After WLS, I relied more upon my bariatric team's weigh-in rather than my own, recognizing that their scales were often more accurate. And the habit has thankfully stuck—I only weigh-in once a week at home, on my own scale, at the same time, with the same clothes on. It's proved reliable.

That said, I have a research scientist friend who says why not look at this like the experts do? They weigh their rats every day, add up the scores over a week, and then divide by seven (the number of days) to get an average score. They do this over time and compare the averages of each week. This averages out the natural fluctuations that occur daily. A good idea if you really can't break the scale-weighing habit. I can't promise it still won't shape your day if you're an "emotional weigher," but it might prove a bit more reliable if you're not.

WILL WEIGHING YOURSELF DAILY HELP YOU STAY ON TRACK?

Stepping on the scale doesn't have to be a scary event for a yearly or monthly doctor's or dietician's visit—and it also doesn't have to be a daily torture ritual at home. There is a happy medium in there.

The Truth. Experts recommend that people weigh themselves once a week, at the same time every week. Weighing yourself every day can have a negative impact on you.

For so many of us, the scale is a source of stress and self-loathing, but it really shouldn't be. Don't think of it as anything other than a compass—something we use when losing weight, to keep us going in the right direction. It tells us what's going on with our bodies so we can effectively modify our regimen to ensure continued weight loss. It's just a tool—no more and no less. So how frequently should you consult it?

Your weight varies throughout the day. Not only does your weight change every day, it also changes at different times throughout a single day, so there's no point in weighing yourself every day—and definitely not multiple times a day. This is because of body fluid fluctuations—you might be retaining water from too much salt consumption, or you may not have gone to the bathroom yet. All of these things affect your weight. The issue with checking *daily* is that minor fluctuations can freak people out—or discourage them from their weight loss efforts.

Instead, take photos and body measurements, and judge yourself by your fitness endurance and how your clothes are fitting.

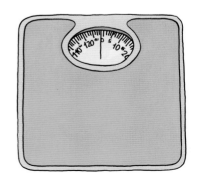

To use the scale effectively, you should weigh yourself once a week. Ideally, you should weigh yourself once a week, at the same time, on the same day of the week, wearing similar clothing, and, most importantly, *on the same scale*. Weighing yourself just once a week will give you a more accurate reading—you'll allow time to actually show weight loss. The number will help you figure out if you need to make adjustments to what you're eating or how you're exercising.

Never weighing yourself is a bad idea. Are you one of those people who doesn't weigh themselves all year, and then finally steps on the scale at their annual physical or bariatric appointment checkup? This isn't the right way to go either! Never weighing yourself and, instead, determining how "healthy" you are by how you feel isn't the best method. To know how healthy you are is to know that number on the scales. If you're in maintenance mode (and not trying to lose weight), I'd still suggest you weigh yourself once a week. Your weight is a total picture of your overall health, and it's good to keep tabs on yourself.

What Your Scale Isn't Telling You

Though weighing regularly can be fun and motivating while losing weight there are many other ways to track your progress.

Here are ways to measure success that go beyond just the scales—your non-scale victories!
1. Take photographs of yourself in the same clothes and in the same location every two or three weeks and create a photo journal.
2. Track your health indicators, like blood pressure, cholesterol, triglycerides, or fasting blood sugar.
3. Keep one pair of each size in pants or skirts and dresses as you lose and compare them to see your progress.
4. Take your measurements every month or two and track your inches lost. Check bust/chest, waist, hips, thighs, ankles, arms, and neck.
5. Log your medicine intake and note how exciting it is when insulin, blood pressure, and other medicines are decreased.

This is proof of the new healthier you!

Dress, Wardrobe, and Beauty Issues

Clothes shopping, love it or loathe it, can be troublesome pre-op and post-op for all sorts of reasons. But I remember the mid-term time being the worst! What do you buy while losing weight after surgery? Do you splash out and treat yourself? Do you just keep wearing the old stuff but cinch it in with a belt? Do you visit the charity shops or beg, steal, and borrow from friends and family? Or do you blithely ignore the changes in your body and deny there's been a change, so you keep wearing the same stuff?

Many of us stall to the point of inertia when thinking about purchasing new clothes—aided with the thinking that we don't know when the weight loss will stop, and don't believe for a long, long time that it won't come back (since it always has in the past).

So it's understandable to be fearful. If you have struggled with weight all your life, shopping is unlikely to be your favorite pastime. And if you are in the process of losing weight, either through a pre-op regimen or as a result of weight loss surgery, buying new clothes for your changing figure can be exciting and frustrating at the same time! Here are some tips and reminders for shopping as you continue on your weight loss journey.

- *Try everything on:* Before you lost weight, you may have avoided the changing room. Now? It's more important than ever to try on everything before you bring it home.

Your body is changing, and your shopping habits need to change with it. What you once pulled off the rack and thought was your size is now, most likely, too big.

- *Be forgiving:* Try to focus on the positives while trying clothing on. Even if you're not the size you ultimately want to be, congratulate yourself on how far you've come. This should also be an incentive to try on some styles that you might not have even considered before.

- *Experiment with new styles and colors:* If you never used to wear a skirt or dress before, why not start wearing them now? Never considered anything "out there" like a bright color? Give it a whirl! Showing off your new body curves is a great way to inspire yourself and create more motivation.

- *Fit your form:* You have a new shape. So why not show it off? Pick new pieces that emphasize your waist or whatever part of your body makes you feel most confident. By choosing pieces that fit well, you can, surprisingly enough, make yourself look thinner. Get rid of those baggy clothes and love the new skin you're in.

- *Have fun:* Take a friend or WLS support buddy shopping with you. They can help you choose some new pieces and give you an honest opinion. They might even nudge you toward stripes!

Plus-Size Fashion Tips for WLS Patients

Many men and women who are plus-size feel that they will never look good until after they have WLS. Not true, and while it may take some searching for an outfit for your larger frame, it is possible to find and put together something when you're larger than average.

Being plus-size does not doom you to a lifetime of dreary dark outfits, tent-like garments, and unfashionable choices; it's just a matter of checking out some of the following ideas:

- *Ladies should start with a firm foundation:* Choosing a good bra, slip, shaper, and tights can make a huge difference in achieving a smooth line under a dress, pants, or skirt. The eye will then go to where it should rather than focus on a bulky undergarment poking through, eliminating muffin tops, bat wings, and all manner of wobbly bits.
- *Wear what you are comfortable in:* No one looks good when they feel uncomfortable, so choose an outfit that makes you feel great. The confidence you display in wearing an outfit you're happy with shines through and enhances your image in countless ways.
- *Make sure that your clothes fit:* It's a myth that larger folk should always choose loose-fitting clothes. Clothes that fit, no matter the size, will always look better than bulky ones that hide your assets. Toss the baggy sweater and look for a figure-shaping alternative.
- *Some age-old advice does hold true:* Darker colors and soft, flowing fabrics are more slimming than brighter and bulky or stiff ones. So opt for classy navy, black, and burgundy, but add a touch of a brighter color for balance and interest.

- *When looking at pattern, keep prints proportionate:* In general terms, the larger you are, the bigger the print or pattern you should choose, since a small print will make you look bigger.
- *Remember to keep accessories proportional, too:* Scale things like belts, jewelry, and scarves to your size. A tiny, delicate item can make you appear larger than you are. Opt instead for bold statement pieces and leave the dainty offerings to the very petite.

Finally, as you're shrinking, don't spend too much on your outfits since they won't usually fit for more than a few weeks after surgery. Consider thrift and charity shops, clothes swapping with other WLS patients, and professional seamstresses to adjust favorite or expensive outfits. A regular wardrobe review is also a must.

If you are feeling really brave, you may want to hire a personal stylist who understands you and what you are looking to achieve, then let them weave their magic for you!

Will I Have Loose Skin After WLS?

If you have watched some extreme makeover programs on TV you may have seen a few patients who have had surgery to "repair" their skin after significant weight loss. This may lead you to wonder if you will experience the same thing after WLS.

Certainly not everyone who loses a lot of weight with WLS will have a problem with "hanging" skin. There are many factors that determine how much loose skin an individual will have after a large weight loss. The most important determinant is probably *age,* as skin naturally becomes less elastic as it ages. The older you are when you lose weight, the less likely your skin will "snap back" to its original shape.

The second most important factor is the *amount of weight loss.* An individual who loses 250 pounds is likely to have more excess skin than someone who loses eighty pounds.

Other less important variables include *complexion, amount of sun exposure* over a lifetime, *heredity,* and whether you are a *smoker.* Fair-skinned people tend to develop more loose skin than darker individuals. Sun worshippers tend to sustain more tissue damage over the years and consequently more loose skin following weight loss. Some people tend to have "better" skin than others of similar complexion and lifestyle. This may be the result of hereditary factors that are not readily apparent. Finally, smoking breaks down collagen, a major component of skin and other structural components of the body. Smokers develop more loose skin than their nonsmoking counterparts.

In other words, having loose skin is one of those things that varies from person to person, and you will not know if it's a problem until it has actually happened.

Most people who lose one hundred pounds or more will usually have a certain degree of excess skin upon reaching their goal weight. This excess is usually in the areas of the body where they used to carry most of their weight, such as the belly. Very rarely does this cause a medical issue, such as skin infections. It is mostly a cosmetic issue and, for many patients, not significant enough to warrant having something done about it.

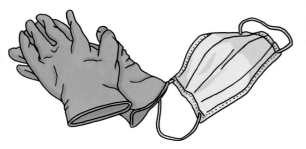

WHAT CAN BE DONE ABOUT IT?

If you have a lot of excess skin that is an issue for you, and you want to have it removed, then you must be referred to a body contouring or body lift surgical specialist for further treatment. This is rarely covered by private health-care insurance and most is funded privately by the individual.

Body contouring consists of a number of cosmetic surgery procedures that lift and tighten skin at various locations of the body (see page 100). Each patient consults with a plastic surgeon to correct their individual problem.

The bottom line? Worrying about the likelihood of having loose skin is no reason to put off losing weight. Losing weight will leave you healthier and will most likely lead to a longer and fuller life.

BODY CONTOURING AND SKIN REMOVAL

Dramatic weight loss is a major accomplishment and has many benefits, especially enhancing your health and self-esteem. However, many people who achieve such weight loss are left with heavy, loose folds of excess skin around their abdomen, thighs, buttocks, breasts, arms, face, and neck. This is because the skin is stretched over a long period of time with the accumulation of fat, and when a large amount of weight is lost, the skin and tissues often lack elasticity and cannot shrink back.

If you have succeeded in losing substantial weight and are left with excess folds of skin, cosmetic surgery may be the only way to reshape your body and complete your weight loss journey.

IS COSMETIC SURGERY FOR ME?

Cosmetic surgery after weight loss is a personal choice. You will need to research the types of cosmetic surgery available and discuss the pros and cons of each with your cosmetic surgeon before making a final decision. You should be mindful of the fact that most cosmetic procedures are major surgery and will carry risks and result in scars. Your consultant will advise you of the risks involved and the possible scars, though the scars are usually hidden in places that are covered by clothes.

Research has shown that patients who undergo reconstructive body contouring plastic surgery following massive weight loss experience significant improvements in their physical function, emotional wellbeing, body image satisfaction, physical well-being, and quality of life.

AM I SUITABLE FOR COSMETIC SURGERY AFTER WLS?

It is recommended that you wait at least eighteen months following your weight loss surgery before having cosmetic surgery, to allow your skin to shrink as much as possible and your weight loss to stabilize. You will also need to be in good health.

If you have a chronic medical condition, such as diabetes or heart disease, your doctor may not recommend cosmetic surgery for you.

If you smoke, you will also need to quit six weeks prior to surgery.

You will also need to be realistic about what to expect from your cosmetic surgery, and you should be aware that your skin will continue to age.

WHAT IS BODY CONTOURING?

Body contouring surgery following major weight loss is the collective name given to the range of cosmetic procedures designed to remove excess sagging fat and skin while improving the shape of the underlying support tissue.

The most problematic areas are the stomach, thighs, buttocks, breasts, upper arms, face, and neck. Your surgeon will work with you and make recommendations about the best strategy to address the areas that are problematic to you. The result of body contouring is a slimmer appearance with smoother contours.

Types of Body Contouring Procedures

Tummy tuck or apronectomy: A tummy tuck (abdominoplasty) removes excess fat and skin from the abdomen and tightens the underlying abdominal muscles. It improves abdominal contours, giving you a flatter and tighter stomach.

An apronectomy, also called a panniculectomy, is a modification of the tummy-tuck for patients who have an overhanging "apron" of skin and fat over the pubic area. It is performed on the lower abdomen below the belly button, and only the surplus skin and fat is removed.

Thigh lift: A thigh lift, as the name suggests, will correct sagging skin on the thighs. It produces more toned thighs that are in proportion to your legs and the rest of your body.

Lower body lift: Many patients find that the majority of weight loss occurs in the buttocks, hips, and thighs. A body lift, also known as a belt lipectomy, removes excess skin from the abdomen, hips, outer thighs, and buttocks.

Breast surgery: Women who have lost substantial weight are often faced with sagging and flattened breasts. Cosmetic breast surgery, including breast uplift and breast enlargement (augmentation) using implants, will remove excess skin while tightening and improving the overall shape of your breasts.

For men, large, sagging breasts can result following weight loss. This is normally treated with a combination of liposuction and skin removal around the breast area called gynecomastia surgery.

Arm lift: An arm lift (brachioplasty) will reduce the fat and excess sagging skin in your upper arm. It tightens and smooths the underlying supportive tissue that defines the shape of the arm.

Face-lift: After weight loss you may notice a sagging of your mid-face, jowls, and neck. A face and neck lift results in a smoother and wrinkle-free face and neck area.

Facelift surgery (rhytidectomy) removes slack facial skin and any unwanted fatty deposits. A neck lift (platysmaplasty) helps to correct sagging skin and wrinkles around the neck and jaw area. With both procedures, the scar is hidden along the front of the ear and in the hair.

Multiple surgeries at once: Your cosmetic surgeon will guide you in deciding whether to have multiple surgeries at once or to space them out over time. Combining a few different procedures at the same time limits the total number of operations and recoveries you will need to have. Most cosmetic surgeries can be combined any way you want. For example, breast reshaping and tummy tuck is a common procedure offered to many patients.

You will need to consider that, the more procedures you combine, the longer you will spend in the operating room. You will also be under anesthesia longer, which may leave you feeling a bit more run down after the surgery.

Hair Loss and Thinning Hair: A Few Tips and Tricks

Hair loss and thinning after bariatric surgery is common, regardless of weight loss surgery procedure.

There are several reasons people lose hair after WLS, and some can be attributed to surgery that involves anesthesia. It is a common side effect.

At any given time, about 90 percent of your hair is in a "growing phase" and the remaining 10 percent is in a "resting phase." After the hair rests for two to three months, it falls out, and new hair grows to replace it.

Anesthesia causes more hair to go into this resting phase than normal (about 30 percent). So it follows that two to three months after surgery, this larger amount of hair falls out. This is usually temporary and the hair does replenish itself in time.

However, there are additional reasons for hair loss after WLS. Rapid loss of weight and reduced nutrition can cause additional hair loss and hair thinning. The best way to minimize this loss is to maximize nutrition.

WLS patients need to aim for about 70 g of protein a day for good nutrition, and supplement their diet with a daily multivitamin. This is essential for all patients, but especially important for gastric bypass patients who cannot absorb all the nutrients they take in as food. Your bariatric team may also recommend a daily dose of calcium citrate, an additional B vitamin complex tablet, and an iron supplement, so follow their guidelines to the letter.

Focusing on getting your nutrition right is the way forward. Most hair loss happens about three to four months after surgery, but hair does grow back to normal after about one year. Gentle shampoos and hair supplements may also help but there is no guaranteed over-the-counter solution.

There is little to alleviate hair loss other than to give the body the chance to repair. But if you do suffer from hair loss, how can you tweak your hair routine to make the most of the hair that you've got? Some of these simple styling tips will add volume and minimize further breakage and loss so that every day becomes, if not a good hair day, a better hair day!

- *Get the right hairstyle:* Too much length can weigh hair down and make it look thinner and flatter. So get a regular cut, trim any split ends, and ask your stylist for a style with layers to add volume.
- *Cut down on hair processing treatments:* Coloring, bleaching, chemical straightening, and chemical curling your hair can weaken the hair shaft and

cause further loss and breakage. If you can't face the thought of not having any, stretch out the time between treatments as much as possible to minimize their detrimental effects.

- *Avoid certain styles:* Don't opt for ponytails, tight buns, braids, or pulled-back headband styles that constantly tug on your hair. This is especially true for those that place stress on the hairline.
- *Limit heat styling to a minimum:* Blow-drying and electric straighteners can do untold damage to weak hair. Blow-drying can literally boil the hair dry! Better to gently towel-dry hair, then use the lowest setting on your hair drier to finish styling. Hair straighteners and curlers should be used on the lowest possible setting for the minimum time.

- *Consider some volumizing products:* Shampoos, conditioners, and other styling products can give your hair a lift by coating the strands of hair to make them look thicker. Use these products sparingly so they don't weigh down your hair and make your scalp more visible. Likewise, only use a modicum of conditioner, hair gel, and hair spray, and just apply these to the ends of your hair rather than near to the scalp.

Looking Good in Photographs

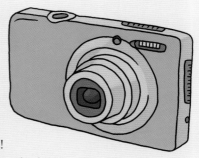

Many WLS patients spend years behind the lens rather than in front of it because of issues with their weight. I know there are some holiday albums of mine where people have queried if I went on the jaunt with the rest of the family. I was conspicuous by my absence in any pictures!

These days, after my surgery and consequent weight loss, I don't automatically volunteer to take the photographs anymore. I push myself forward, so that I can appear in photographs like the rest of my family, friends, and associates.

But, that said, we all know that facial expression can make a big difference in how photos turn out—you can look your best or you can look "not so hot." Pose and poise can make or break a picture and make it a winner or loser. Here are some tricks to help you loosen up and look your natural best.

- The number-one celebrity photo trick is to put one hand on your hip. Not sure? Well check out your latest celeb magazine and see how many A-listers adopt this position! This pose reminds you to keep your shoulders back and not to slouch. It also helps to define your waist if you're wearing something loose. Just remember to keep your fingers together so that you don't have jazz hands.

- Say cheese by all means but if you've been smiling for a long time, close your eyes for a few seconds or look down and then up at the camera—the brief pause will help you to avoid having a glassy-eyed stare.
- If you're being photographed while standing, face the camera and turn your body at an angle. Stand with one leg slightly in front of the other, feet pointed slightly outward. You'll look taller and thinner. Don't stand with your legs apart or you'll look like a football player! Practice in front of a full-length mirror so that you'll feel comfortable when it's picture time.

If you're pre-op or early post-op, try out these tips when taking your "before and after" pics in the record of your weight loss journey.

Some Cures for the Curse of Summer Chafing

Every year, when summer comes around, the problem of chafing rears its ugly head. In cool weather, it's not a problem: fleshy bits glide smoothly past each other. But as it gets warmer—and we start to perspire—the tops of our thighs can stick together. The resulting friction causes what's colloquially known as "chub rub."

It may sound amusing, but anyone who's suffered the stinging, burning, bright-red rash that makes it painful to walk will tell you it's anything but.

You could wear pants to stop your thighs rubbing against each other, but many of us, especially if we have lost a lot of weight, would rather spend the summer in pretty dresses. So what other options are there?

- *Balms:* These moisturize the skin and help it slide rather than rub. There are some basic ones, but also consider baby formulas and those for athletes (especially cyclists).
- *Friction-free powders:* Thinner than ordinary talc, they help the skin glide. Some have a medicated formula.
- *Undergarment shorts:* Ideal if you don't mind the additional bulk, but watch out for gusts of wind that may reveal your "cure."
- *Bandalette garters:* These 6-inch (15 cm) stretchy lace garters are a pretty option and look more intentional as a deliberate fashion statement than shorts. With silicone at the top and the bottom, they also stay in place. They are available in many styles from plain to lacy and in many colors.

PART TWO

———

The Recipes

How to Use This Cookbook

The recipes that follow have been specifically developed and designed to help you at every stage after WLS. There are recipes for every stage: Fluids, Soft Foods, and Foods for Life. They have been color-coded Red, Yellow, and Green to make identification and selection easy.

Many can of course also be used in pre-op stages (though not for the liver-reducing diet—see page 22). They are also intended for you to eat and share with friends and family. You don't need to eat your meals apart from others.

If the recipe has been color-coded as suitable for your eating stage, it can be considered for your eating plan, although in some cases the WLS portion may need to be puréed or mashed before serving.

People's tolerances vary greatly, so while an ingredient or recipe may be recommended for a specific stage of your diet progression, only you will know what you can tolerate and when.

You will find a nutritional analysis breakdown in every recipe that includes calories, protein, carbohydrates, and fats. All analyses are based on the normal or average portion size, unless otherwise stated.

At the top of each recipe, you'll find a button with the WLS portion size, to make it easy to cook and eat as a family. For example, if the recipe serves 4 and the WLS portion is suggested at ½–1, the recipe would serve 4–8 WLS portions.

WLS PORTION: ½–1

WHAT DO YOU MEAN BY NORMAL AND WLS PORTION?

A normal portion is what a non-WLS person would eat and the WLS portion is often a fraction of this. Both are given so that you can still eat as a family and not always as a "lone" diner.

So for example, if a recipe says it serves four but the WLS portion is suggested at half, then the whole recipe would serve eight WLS portions.

In order to calculate your macros (nutritional analysis), you would need to also halve the quantities stated for calories, protein, carbs, and fat, since this is given for the normal-size portion.

The WLS portion size is flexible and has been based upon testing at my website, Bariatric Cookery, and sampling among a number of patients with different surgeries. Undoubtedly they vary from surgical type, length out of surgery, gender, and other variables, but they serve as a general guide.

Don't be afraid to be flexible with these recipes, food suggestions, and portion recommendations. For example, if you find beef indigestible, use turkey or chicken instead. If you find the portion size always a little on the larger side, downgrade across the board. If you dislike artificial sweeteners, use a substitute. If you don't like a seasoning, try another. Make this new way of eating work for you.

Recipes are also coded for suitability for freezing with this symbol ✱ and for vegetarians with this Ⓥ.

For the record, measuring-spoon measurements unless otherwise stated are level; eggs unless otherwise stated are medium; and when a microwave is used, it has a power output of 900 watts.

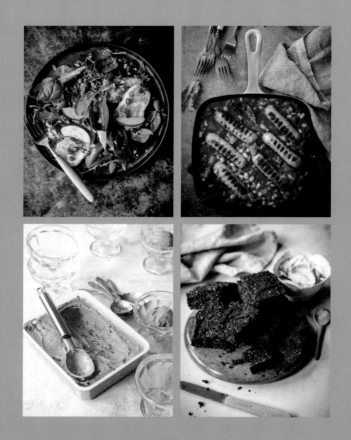

Recipes

—

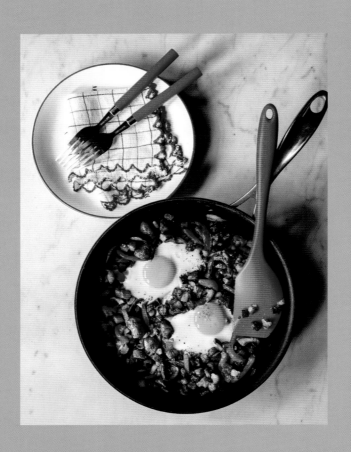

Breakfasts
and Brunches

Creamiest Vanilla Oatmeal with Berry Compote

This elevated oatmeal is made with quark, rather than just milk, and is served with a super berry compote, producing a sublime breakfast bowl.

○ ● ●		SERVES **2**		**V**
PER PORTION (using honey):	CALORIES **261**	PROTEIN **10.2 g**	CARBOHYDRATE **46.2 g**	FAT **3.3 g**

4 ounces (125 g) fresh or frozen mixed berries (such as blueberries, strawberries, and raspberries)

4 teaspoons honey, or other sweetener of your choice

1 cup (75 g) rolled oats

4 ounces (125 g) vanilla quark, or plain quark flavored with vanilla extract to taste

1. **To make the compote,** place the berries and honey in a small pan and gently bring to a boil. If you're using a granulated sweetener, add 1 to 2 tablespoons water. Reduce the heat and simmer gently until the berries have softened. Remove from the heat and allow to cool.

2. **To make the oatmeal,** place the oats and 1½ cups (375 ml) water in a nonstick pan and bring to a boil. Reduce the heat and simmer over low heat for 4 to 5 minutes, stirring occasionally until the mixture has thickened.

3. Add the quark and stir until the mixture is smooth and creamy. Remove from the heat and spoon into bowls. Serve immediately, topped with the prepared compote.

VARIATION **Bircher-Style Oatmeal and Berry Pot:** Prepare the compote as above. Mix the oats with the water and quark and divide between two jars. Top each with half of the berry mixture. Screw on the lids, then chill overnight. Mix the berries into the oat mixture and eat.

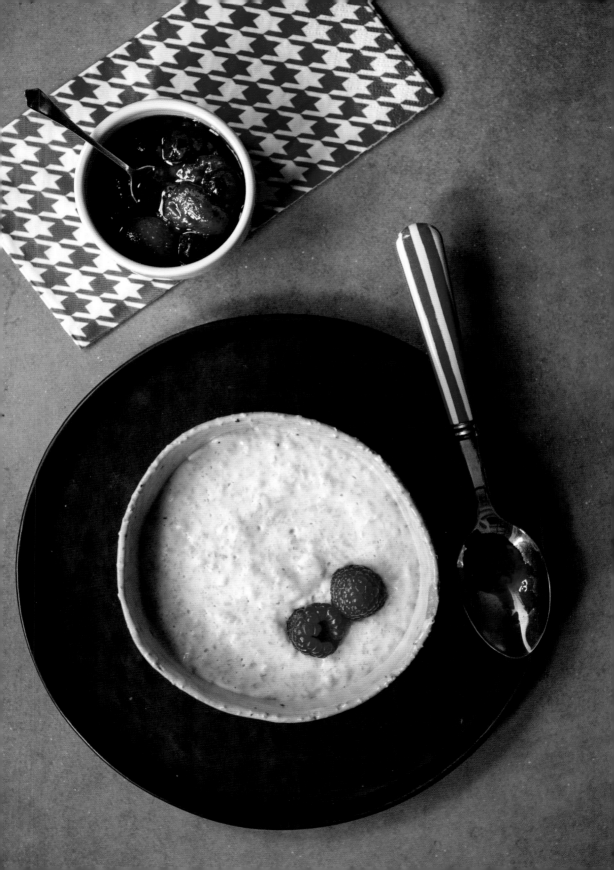

Spiced Oat, Apple, and Coconut Smoothie Bowl

Smoothie bowls have gained huge popularity recently and are ideal for bariatric post–ops. I make mine with oats and yogurt as the base but go wild with a variety of toppings from fruits and nuts to seeds and spices. Early post–ops may want to go easy with their choice of toppings until they know they can tolerate them but once confirmed, the choice is almost limitless.

○ ● ●		SERVES 2		Ⓥ
PER PORTION:	CALORIES **320**	PROTEIN **15.3 g**	CARBOHYDRATE **41.7 g**	FAT **9.9 g**

²/₃ cup (75 g) old-fashioned rolled oats

²/₃ cup (175 g) fat-free Greek yogurt

1 large banana, sliced and frozen

¼ cup plus 2 tablespoons (90 ml) coconut water, chilled

Pinch of salt

Vanilla extract, to taste

1 apple, cored and chopped

1 tablespoon flaked coconut, or fresh shaved coconut

1 tablespoon mixed seeds and nuts

1. Purée the oats with the yogurt, banana, coconut water, salt and vanilla extract to taste in a blender until smooth.
2. Pour into bowls and top with the apple, coconut, and mixed seeds and nuts to serve.

Clementine, Cranberry, and Pecan Bircher Muesli

This colorful, fresh fruit breakfast or brunch dish can be made the night before, keeping things very simple for the next day. Change it up by using sliced oranges, walnuts, and other berries as liked and in season.

○ ○ ●		SERVES **4**		**V**
PER PORTION:	CALORIES **293**	PROTEIN **11.8 g**	CARBOHYDRATE **46.5 g**	FAT **6.7 g**

1²/₃ cups (150 g) old-fashioned rolled oats

1 apple, cored and grated

²/₃ cup (150 ml) low-fat milk

2 teaspoons pumpkin seeds

½ cup (125 ml) orange juice

2 ounces (50 g) dried cranberries

½ teaspoon ground cinnamon

1½ teaspoons maple or sugar-free fruit syrup

¾ cup (200 g) fat-free plain Greek yogurt

1 clementine, peeled and segmented

8 toasted pecans

1. In a bowl, mix the oats with the apple, milk, pumpkin seeds, orange juice, half the cranberries, cinnamon, syrup, and yogurt, mixing well. Cover and leave to soak for at least 3 hours or ideally overnight in the refrigerator.

2. When ready to serve, spoon the muesli into bowls and top with the clementine segments and pecans. Scatter the remaining cranberries on top to serve.

Granola and Fruit Breakfast Tartlets

These delicious and healthy breakfast tarts, made with a granola crust, look as good as they taste. Change it up by using different granolas, prepared fresh fruit in season, as well as changing the yogurt variety or using quark instead.

○ ○ ●		MAKES 4		Ⓥ
PER TARTLET (using berries):	CALORIES **277**	PROTEIN **12.4 g**	CARBOHYDRATE **26 g**	FAT **13.8 g**

1½ cups (100 g) low-sugar granola mix, or rolled oats

¼ cup (25 g) mixed chopped nuts

2 tablespoons mixed seeds

1 tablespoon dried or flaked coconut

1 tablespoon coconut or other oil

2 tablespoons sugar-free syrup, agave syrup, or honey

1¼ cups (250 g) fat-free Greek yogurt

2 teaspoons sweetener (optional)

Handful of berries, or about 6 ounces (175 g) prepared fresh fruit

Mint sprigs, to decorate

1. Preheat the oven to 350°F (180°C). Lightly grease 4 mini loose-bottomed tartlet pans.
2. Place the granola or oats, nuts, seeds, coconut, and coconut oil in a food processor and pulse to form a crumb-like consistency. Melt the coconut oil, if necessary (in the microwave for just a few seconds), then mix with the syrup, agave, or honey. Add to the granola mixture and pulse again to combine. Remove and divide among the tartlet pans. Make a crust for the tartlets by firmly pressing down on the bottom and sides of the pans so that you form a smooth base. Place on a baking sheet. Bake for 8 to 10 minutes or until the crust begins to brown— take care not to overcook, since the mixture burns easily. Remove from the oven and let cool in their pans.
3. To serve, remove the tartlets from their pans and place on a serving plate. Mix the yogurt with the sweetener, if using. Divide among the granola crusts and top with fruit to serve, garnished with mint sprigs.

Breakfast Protein Pancakes

WLS
PORTION:
1

These thick and soft protein pancakes can be made with low-fat milk if you prefer a less dense texture. They are lovely with low-sugar preserves, fruit (like sliced banana and berries), or simply drizzled with a little low-sugar syrup.

○ ◐ ●		MAKES **4**		**V**
PER PANCAKE (using egg whites):	CALORIES **64**	PROTEIN **8.3 g**	CARBOHYDRATE **2.5 g**	FAT **1.5 g**

1 egg or 2 egg whites

2 tablespoons coconut flour (or whole wheat flour, if preferred)

¼ cup (50 g) low-fat Greek yogurt

1 ounce (25 g) low-fat, low-sugar vanilla protein powder

½ teaspoon baking powder

Low-fat cooking spray

1. **To make the pancake batter,** mix the egg or egg whites with the coconut flour, yogurt, protein powder, and baking powder until smooth.
2. Spray a large frying pan with low-fat cooking spray. Heat, then spoon the pancake batter in to make 4 small pancakes.
3. Cook for 2 to 3 minutes, until browned on the underside, then flip over and cook for a further 1 to 2 minutes.
4. Serve warm with preserves, fruit, extra yogurt, or syrup, as desired.

Protein-Laden Eggs Benedict

This version of eggs Benedict is just as luxurious as the usual one with a buttery hollandaise sauce. It works by replacing some of the butter with high-protein plain yogurt, which results in a dish that is higher in protein and lower in fat—but just as delicious! High-protein yogurt refers to any yogurt with a protein content of around 11 g per 100 g—Greek-style is a good choice. Serve over toasted bread, if desired.

○ ◐ ●	SERVES 2	Ⓥ		
PER PORTION (without toast):	CALORIES **270**	PROTEIN **15.3 g**	CARBOHYDRATE **2.9 g**	FAT **21.8 g**

⅓ cup (100 g) high-protein, low-fat yogurt

1 teaspoon mustard

1 teaspoon white wine vinegar

Squeeze of lemon juice

2 tablespoons butter

2 egg yolks

2 poached eggs

Toasted bread, to serve (optional)

1. **To make the sauce,** mix the yogurt with the mustard, vinegar, and lemon juice in a bowl.
2. Melt the butter in a small pan, turn the heat down as low as possible and add the yogurt mixture, mixing well. Slowly beat in the egg yolks with a whisk and heat until warm but not hot enough to curdle. Turn off the heat and leave to stand while poaching the eggs.
3. Poach the eggs and place on top of a slice of toasted bread, if desired. Spoon over the prepared sauce and serve immediately.

Fried Egg on Parmesan "Toast"

WLS PORTION: ½–1

Few can resist "egg on toast" for breakfast since it makes for a speedy start to the day. But many WLS patients shun bread or can't tolerate it and miss out on this staple. Here's an alternative solution—a fried egg cooked atop a lacy, crunchy Parmesan cheese crisp—ingenious! It's also good with crispy bacon and a slice of avocado.

○ ○ ●		SERVES 1		**Ⓥ**
PER PORTION (with salad greens and tomatoes):	CALORIES **198**	PROTEIN **16.4 g**	CARBOHYDRATE **3 g**	FAT **13.3 g**

¼ cup (25 g) grated Parmesan cheese

1 egg

Salt and freshly ground black pepper

Salad greens and halved baby tomatoes, to serve (optional)

1. Heat a small nonstick frying pan over medium heat until hot (you can test by dropping in a little cheese—it should sizzle when ready to cook).

2. Add the cheese in an even layer and quickly smooth it out to slightly larger than the size of a fried egg. Heat until the cheese begins to bubble, about 30 to 50 seconds.

3. Crack the egg directly on top of the cheese (or crack into a cup and then slide onto the cheese). Cook until the edges are just set, about 2 minutes. Cover and continue cooking until the white is set but the yolk is still soft and runny, about 1½ minutes. The cheese crisp should be crispy and golden.

4. Season with salt and pepper, run a spatula around the edge of the cheese crisp to loosen, then lift to transfer to a plate to serve.

5. Serve plain or with a few salad greens and halved tomatoes, or with your favorite breakfast/brunch items, like bacon, sausage, or mushrooms.

Veggie and Egg Breakfast Sizzle

WLS PORTION: ½–1

Eggs make a most nutritious breakfast dish for the WLS patient—lightly scrambled, boiled, made into an omelet, baked, souffléd, or cooked with other ingredients to make a tortilla. They offer great variety and a speedy solution to breakfast eating. This dish can be on the table in ten minutes and, when served with toast, makes a substantial breakfast or brunch.

○ ○ ●		SERVES 4		Ⓥ
PER PORTION:	CALORIES **145**	PROTEIN **11.9 g**	CARBOHYDRATE **6.7 g**	FAT **7.9 g**

Low-fat cooking spray

1 small onion, chopped

3 zucchini, chopped

5 ounces (150 g) mushrooms, sliced

1 red bell pepper, cored, seeded, and chopped

2 tablespoons chopped fresh basil

Salt and freshly ground black pepper

4 large eggs

1. Generously spray a large nonstick frying pan with low-fat cooking spray. Heat, add the onion, zucchini, mushrooms, and bell pepper, and cook over a high heat for 4 to 6 minutes, stirring until golden and softened. Stir in the basil and salt and pepper.

2. Make 4 hollows in the mixture, then crack an egg into each. Reduce the heat, cover the pan, and cook for about 3 minutes, until the eggs are cooked and set to your liking.

3. Serve immediately with a little toast, if tolerated.

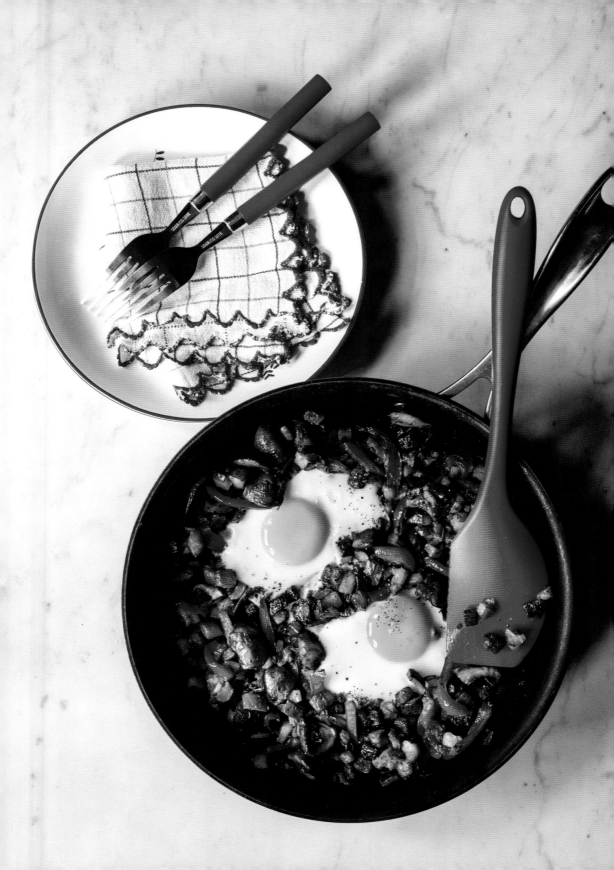

Scrambled Omelet with Cheese and Cherry Tomatoes

WLS PORTION: ½

This is a breakfast dish that I frequently make and eat. I sometimes use soft sun-dried tomatoes (snipped into pieces) instead of the cherry tomatoes. In the early days, I could only eat a quarter to a half portion and so would save the remainder to eat for lunch with a salad. It can be reheated quickly in the microwave but is equally good cold.

	SERVES 1			V
PER PORTION:	CALORIES **268**	PROTEIN **20.6 g**	CARBOHYDRATE **2.9 g**	FAT **19.4 g**

2 teaspoons light butter or low-fat spread

2 eggs, lightly beaten

2 tablespoons skim or low-fat milk

Salt and freshly ground black pepper

6 cherry tomatoes, quartered

1 tablespoon grated reduced-fat hard cheese

Snipped fresh chives, to garnish

1. Heat a small nonstick omelet or frying pan. Add the butter or low-fat spread to melt.
2. Mix the eggs with the milk and salt and pepper. Pour into the pan and cook for about 1 minute to set slightly.
3. Stir or scramble briefly, add the tomatoes and cook for a further 1 to 2 minutes until the mixture is just set.
4. Sprinkle with the cheese and chives.
5. Fold the omelet to serve.

Cheesy Jello Pots

WLS PORTION: ½–1

I first made this mixture with yogurt as a dessert but then realized if I used cottage cheese instead of the yogurt, it would make a great breakfast dish. You can vary the flavor of the Jello to add variety and even stir in some berries before leaving it to set. These mousses can be made well ahead and will keep for three to four days in the refrigerator. You can also use quark or fat-free Greek yogurt instead of the cottage cheese, if preferred.

○ ◐ ●		SERVES **4**		**V**
PER PORTION:	CALORIES **74**	PROTEIN **13.2 g**	CARBOHYDRATE **3.1 g**	FAT **1 g**

1-ounce packet (23 g) sugar-free Jello

1½ cups (300 g) low-fat cottage cheese

1. Dissolve the Jello in 1 cup (250 ml) boiling water, stirring well until clear. Allow to cool slightly.
2. Place the cottage cheese and cooled (but still liquid) Jello in a blender and blend until smooth.
3. Divide among 4 jars, glasses, or small ramekins and chill until set, about 2 to 3 hours.

Breakfast Scones

I make these scones on the weekend or when we have people stay over, since they happily straddle the divide between breakfast and lunch. They are also wonderfully time-tolerant for late risers. You can make a vegetarian option by replacing the bacon with finely chopped scallions.

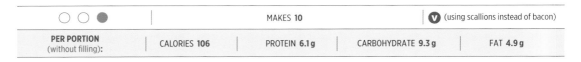

○ ○ ●	MAKES **10**	**V** (using scallions instead of bacon)

PER PORTION (without filling):	CALORIES **106**	PROTEIN **6.1 g**	CARBOHYDRATE **9.3 g**	FAT **4.9 g**

Low-fat cooking spray

1 cup (100 g) mushrooms, chopped

1¼ cups (125 g) all-purpose flour

1¼ teaspoons baking powder

¼ cup (50 g) light butter or low-fat spread

5 ounces (150 g) lean bacon or turkey bacon, grilled or broiled and chopped

½ cup (50 g) grated reduced-fat hard cheese

½ cup (100 ml) low-fat milk

Low-fat soft cheese, ham, and sliced tomatoes, to fill, as desired

1. Preheat the oven to 425°F (220°C). Grease a baking sheet with low-fat cooking spray.
2. Generously spray a small pan with low-fat cooking spray. Heat, add the mushrooms, and cook for 4 to 5 minutes, until golden. Let cool.
3. Mix the flour with baking powder in a large bowl. Rub in the butter or spread until the mixture resembles fine bread crumbs.
4. Stir in the bacon, mushrooms, and half of the cheese. Mix in the milk to form a soft dough.
5. Roll out the dough on a lightly floured surface to ¾-inch (2 cm) thickness. Stamp out rounds with a 2½-inch (6 cm) round cutter. The mixture will make about 10 scones.
6. Place on the baking sheet and sprinkle with the remaining cheese.
7. Bake for 10 to 15 minutes, until cooked and golden.
8. Serve warm or cold, filled with low-fat cheese, ham, and sliced tomatoes, if desired.

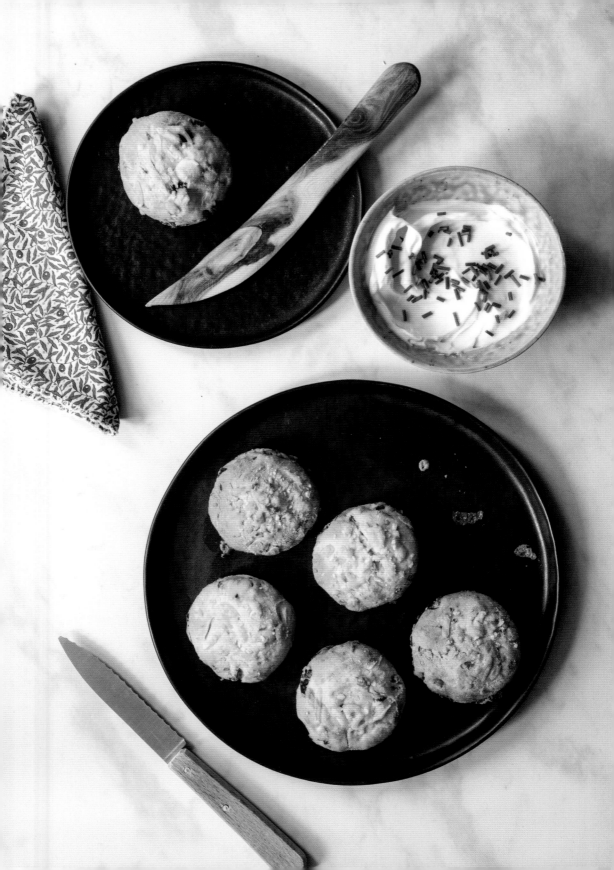

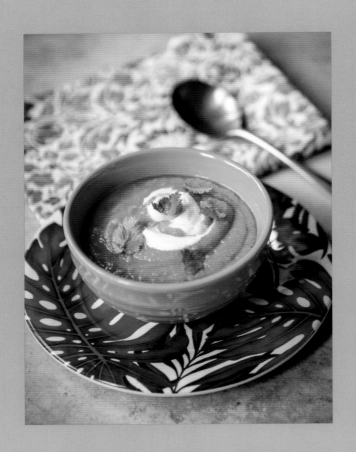

Lunches and Light Meals

Apple and Lentil Soup

Soups are often the mainstay (along with smoothies and shakes) of the Red (fluid) stage of eating, but so many are full of sugar, modified starch, and synthetic ingredients. I urge you to make your own, and this is a great one to start with. It's basically a lentil and carrot soup with the addition of apples (for natural sweetness), some spices, and just a dash of coconut milk to give it a more exciting flavor. You'll make this soup again and again, and it will become a permanent staple in your WLS recipe repertoire.

● ● ●		SERVES 6		Ⓥ		✱
PER PORTION:		CALORIES **172**	PROTEIN **8.5 g**	CARBOHYDRATE **26.3 g**		FAT **4 g**

½ teaspoon crushed red pepper flakes

2 teaspoons cumin seeds

Low-fat cooking spray

1 pound (450 g) carrots, peeled and cut into small pieces

2 cooking apples (about 1 pound/450 g), peeled, cored, and roughly chopped

1 stalk celery, finely sliced

⅔ cup (125 g) red lentils

Generous 3 cups (750 ml) hot vegetable stock

1 cup (250 ml) light or reduced-fat coconut milk

Salt and freshly ground black pepper

¼ cup (65 g) fat-free Greek yogurt, to serve

¼ cup (15 g) chopped fresh cilantro, to garnish (optional)

1. Heat a large pan and add the crushed red pepper flakes and cumin seeds. Fry for 1 to 2 minutes, until they release their aroma and pop around the pan. Remove half the flakes and seeds and set aside.

2. Generously spray the pan with low-fat cooking spray, heat, and then add the carrots, apples, and celery. Cook for 5 minutes, then add the lentils, stock, and coconut milk. Bring to a simmer, cover, and cook for 15 minutes, or until the carrots and lentils are tender.

3. Purée the soup in a blender until smooth, then season to taste with salt and pepper.

4. To serve, ladle the soup into bowls, top with a swirl of yogurt, and garnish with the cilantro, if desired. Scatter with the reserved toasted spices (or omit if you prefer a less spicy soup).

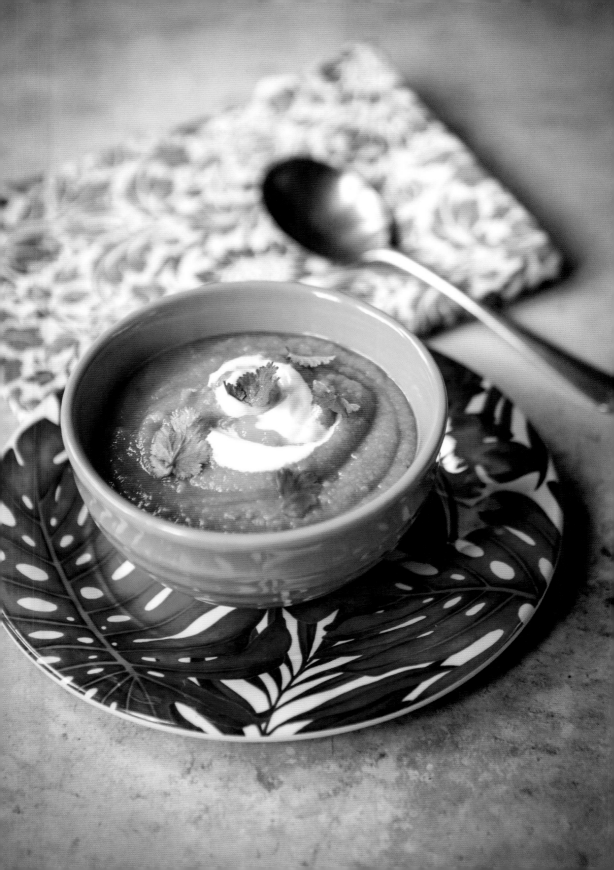

Sweet Potato, Ginger, and Carrot Soup

WLS PORTION: ½–1

There are plenty of times when I want something sweet, warm, and comforting, especially during the winter months. This soup is one of my default recipes, with undertones of ginger and cumin. It's a great recipe for vegetarians and vegans, too (without the yogurt topping), and freezes beautifully. It's well worth making a batch for a soothing cupful anytime.

	SERVES 6		Ⓥ	✳
PER PORTION:	CALORIES **150**	PROTEIN **2.8 g**	CARBOHYDRATE **33 g**	FAT **1.8 g**

Low-fat cooking spray

2 pounds (900 g) sweet potatoes, peeled and chopped

1 pound (450 g) carrots, peeled and chopped

1-inch (2.5 cm) piece ginger, peeled and grated

1 teaspoon ground cumin

6 cups (1.4 L) vegetable stock

Salt and freshly ground black pepper

Fat-free plain yogurt, snipped fresh chives, and grated carrot, to garnish (optional)

1. Generously spray a large nonstick pan with low-fat cooking spray. Heat, add the sweet potatoes, carrots, ginger, and cumin, and cook over high heat for about 10 minutes, stirring occasionally, until starting to brown.
2. Add the stock and salt and pepper, bring to a boil, cover, reduce heat, and simmer for about 40 minutes, until the vegetables are tender.
3. Purée in a blender until smooth. Return to the pan and reheat until hot.
4. Ladle into warmed bowls or cups and top with a swirl of plain yogurt, a sprinkling of chives, and a little grated carrot, if desired.

"Get the Glow" Lentil Soup

WLS PORTION: ½

This is one of my most favorite soups, because it sings with flavor. It's easy to cook, has a spicy but not "hot" flavor, freezes well, and suits all stages of eating (excluding clear liquid) after surgery. I enjoy it with a slice of protein bread, but it's filling enough without.

● ● ●	SERVES 6	ⓥ	✱
PER PORTION:	CALORIES **192**	PROTEIN **8.1 g**	CARBOHYDRATE **23 g**	FAT **7.7 g**

Low-fat cooking spray

2 large onions, chopped

1 garlic clove, crushed

2 teaspoons ground turmeric

¼ teaspoon ground cardamom

1½ teaspoons ground cumin

½ teaspoon ground cinnamon

One 14-ounce (400 g) can diced tomatoes

One 14-ounce (400 g) can reduced-fat coconut milk

¾ cup (140 g) red lentils

3¾ cups (900 ml) vegetable stock

Salt and freshly ground black pepper

1. Spray a large pan with low-fat cooking spray and heat. Add the onions and garlic and cook over low heat until softened, about 5 minutes.
2. Add the turmeric, cardamom, cumin, and cinnamon, and mix well. Cook for 1 minute.
3. Add the tomatoes and their juice, coconut milk, lentils, stock, and salt and pepper, mixing well. Bring to a low boil.
4. Simmer uncovered for about 20 to 25 minutes, until the lentils are cooked and tender and the soup has thickened.
5. Check and adjust the seasoning and serve hot or warm.

NOTE: Purée in a blender until smooth for the early stages of eating—Fluid (Red) and Soft Food (Yellow)—after surgery.

Crustless Quiche with Tuna

I developed this basic recipe for those who, post-surgery, can't tolerate pastry or need to monitor carefully their carb and fat intake. It is very, very versatile as you can add almost anything to the mix (I've used tuna below as a guide) but I frequently use leftover roasted vegetables from Sunday lunch, stir-fry vegetables from a supper dish, remains from a deli platter, or surplus mushrooms, tomatoes, bacon, and sausages from a cooked breakfast. It is perfect to repurpose any leftover food.

THE BASICS: All you need are some staples like meat, vegetables, flaked fish, or a vegetarian mixture; seasonings, and ideally a bit of cheese, for flavoring. For an 8-inch (20 cm) quiche dish, I use 4 eggs either mixed with about ½ cup (100 ml) skim or low-fat milk, or scant 1 cup (200 g) low-fat cottage cheese and a good handful or two of my chosen staples. Simply mix all together (or follow the exact instructions below) and bake at 375°F (190°C) for 25 to 30 minutes. You can make individual mini quiches from the same mixture (and swap the fillings for variety) and bake for about 15 minutes. This will make about 12 mini quiche.

Here's a tuna version to give you a little more detail.

			SERVES 6		
PER PORTION:	CALORIES 142	PROTEIN 21 g	CARBOHYDRATE 3.3 g	FAT 5 g

Low-fat cooking spray

One 14-ounce (400 g) can tuna in water, drained and flaked

4 eggs, beaten

Scant 1 cup (200 g) low-fat cottage cheese with chives

6 scallions, chopped

Salt and freshly ground black pepper

2 tomatoes, sliced

2 teaspoons mixed dried herbs (optional)

1. Preheat the oven to 375°F (190°C). Generously spray an 8-inch (20 cm) quiche dish with low-fat cooking spray.
2. Place the tuna in the dish and spread out evenly.
3. Mix the eggs with the cottage cheese, scallions, and salt and pepper. Pour over the tuna mixture to cover evenly.
4. Top with the sliced tomatoes and sprinkle with the dried herbs, if using.
5. Bake for 25 to 30 minutes, until set and golden.
6. Serve hot with vegetables, cold with salad, or pack into a lunch box for a portable meal.

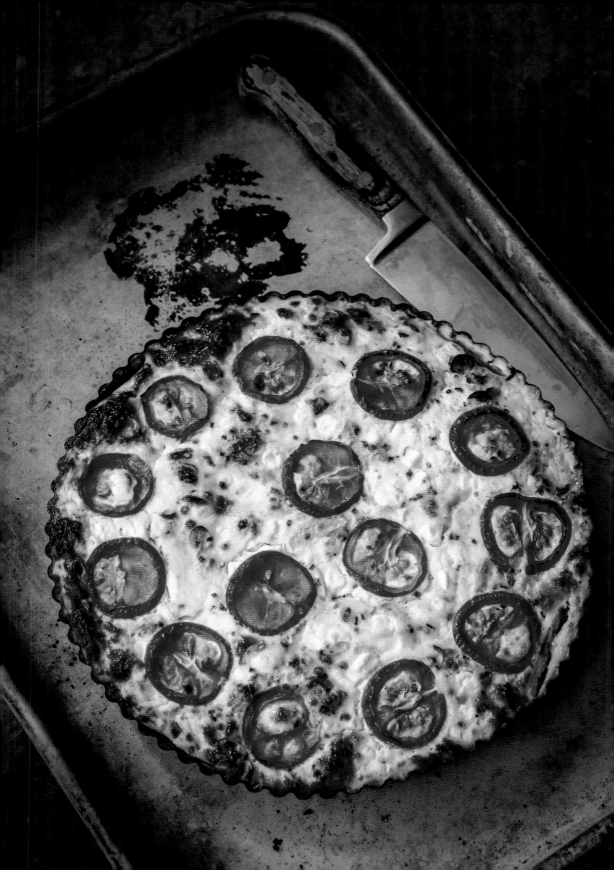

Bariatric Tortilla Pizza

Here's a pizza recipe that I have been making over the years and keep coming back to in spite of trying cauliflower and chickpea flour variations. Why? Well, it's very easy to prepare, unlike the others, is generally lighter for a lunch, and can be on the table quicker than the pizza man delivers! The secret is in using a tortilla for the base—I opt for a low-carb one and load up with protein-rich toppings, though I make sure not to add them too far in advance, or it can go a bit soggy. The other secret is to eat it straight from the oven. I've given a basic recipe below, but feel free to adjust and add your own favorite pizza toppings.

○ ○ ● | SERVES **2**

PER PORTION:	CALORIES **245**	PROTEIN **22 g**	CARBOHYDRATE **11.9 g**	FAT **12.3 g**

1 low-carb whole wheat tortilla

2 tablespoons tomato paste, or thick tomato salsa

2 ounces (50 g) chopped cooked ham, or crumbled bacon

6 cherry tomatoes, halved

4 ounces (125 g) reduced-fat mozzarella, thinly sliced

6 olives or anchovy fillets

2 teaspoons chopped fresh herbs (optional)

Salt and freshly ground black pepper

1 teaspoon grated Parmesan cheese

A few sprigs fresh basil or arugula leaves, to serve (optional)

1. Preheat the oven to 375°F (190°C).

2. Lightly grease a baking sheet or line with parchment paper. Place the tortilla on top.

3. Spread the tomato paste or salsa evenly over the tortilla and top with the ham or bacon. Add the tomatoes, mozzarella, olives or anchovy fillets, and herbs, if using. Season with salt and pepper and sprinkle on the Parmesan.

4. Bake for 10 minutes. Top with basil sprigs or scatter with arugula to serve. Cut into wedges to serve with salad, if desired.

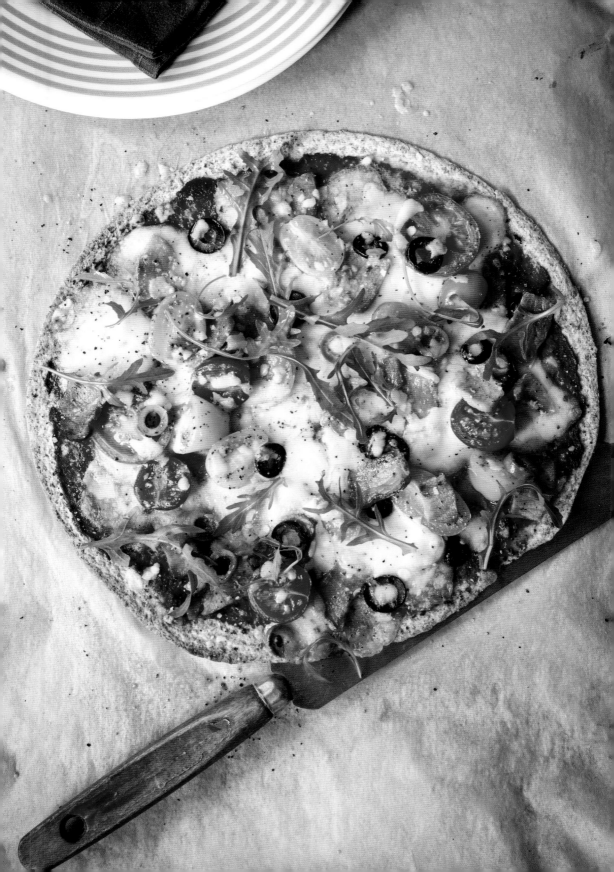

Tomatoes on Chickpea Purée

Here's a light meal-replacement for tomatoes on toast, which will be most welcome at the Soft Food (Yellow) stage after surgery. The chickpeas also give a great protein boost.

	SERVES **2**	Ⓥ
PER PORTION:	CALORIES **190**	PROTEIN **10.8 g**	CARBOHYDRATE **28.7 g**	FAT **3.7 g**

One 14-ounce (400 g) can chickpeas

6 to 8 cardamom pods, crushed and seeds removed

Salt and freshly ground black pepper

3 tomatoes, thickly sliced

Low-fat cooking spray

1 teaspoon honey or sugar-free fruit syrup

2 tablespoons chopped fresh parsley

Lemon juice, to taste

1. Drain the chickpeas, reserving the liquid. Set 2 tablespoons of the whole chickpeas aside and place the remainder in a food processor. Add 5 tablespoons of the reserved liquid, the cardamom seeds, and salt and pepper. Purée until smooth. Place in a small pan and heat very gently while preparing the tomatoes.

2. Generously spray a nonstick frying pan with low-fat cooking spray, heat, and add the tomatoes. Season with salt and pepper, and cook on both sides, until slightly softened.

3. Spoon the warm chickpea purée onto serving plates and top with the cooked tomatoes and reserved whole chickpeas.

4. Add 2 tablespoons of the reserved chickpea liquid to the frying pan with the honey, parsley, and a squeeze of lemon juice, and heat until bubbly. Drizzle over the tomatoes to serve.

Lentils with Roasted Tomatoes
and Horseradish Cottage Cheese

WLS PORTION: ½

The Soft Food (Yellow) stage of eating can be very challenging, but this simple lunch dish is perfect. It's made with soft-cooked lentils, roasted tomatoes, and cottage cheese, but can be "beefed" up at later stages with additional protein in the form of shredded cooked poultry or flaked fish. For speed and convenience, I've made it extra easy to prepare by using a vacuum pouch of ready-cooked beluga or French puy lentils but you can, of course, cook your own. Likewise, vary or omit the herbs if you're not keen on lemon thyme and change the horseradish flavoring in the cottage cheese, as desired (perhaps for something milder, like chives).

○ ● ●		SERVES 2		Ⅴ
PER PORTION:	CALORIES **305**	PROTEIN **27.2 g**	CARBOHYDRATE **34.2 g**	FAT **4.8 g**

1 cup (200 g) low-fat cottage cheese

1 tablespoon prepared horseradish

12 ounces (350 g) cherry tomatoes

2 garlic cloves, crushed

Salt and freshly ground black pepper

2 tablespoons chopped fresh thyme (optional)

Low-fat cooking spray

8 ounces (250 g) vacuum pack beluga or puy lentils

A few sprigs lemon thyme, to garnish (optional)

1. Preheat the oven to 400°F (200°C).
2. Mix the cottage cheese with the horseradish and set aside.
3. Halve the cherry tomatoes and place on a baking sheet. Sprinkle with the garlic, season with salt and pepper, and scatter over the thyme, if used. Spray with a little low-fat cooking spray, then roast for 10 to 15 minutes, until softened.
4. Just before the tomatoes are cooked, microwave the lentils to reheat (or follow the package instructions), about 1 minute, and tip into a bowl.
5. Add the tomatoes with their juices and very gently mix together.
6. Spoon onto a serving plate and top with the prepared cottage cheese. Garnish with a few sprigs of fresh lemon thyme, if desired. This is good served hot or cold.

Energy Bowl

WLS PORTION: ½

I just adore bowls of grains, fruit, seeds, nuts and cheese—not only because they are colorful and inviting but also infinitely versatile. I use whatever is in season but also what I have in my cupboard. Feel free, therefore, to adapt this recipe to your own tastes. The quinoa in the recipe below hasn't been flavored in any additional way (the fruit adds enough, I think) but you could add a little fat-free dressing, if desired.

	○ ○ ●	SERVES **4**	Ⓥ	
PER PORTION:	CALORIES **298**	PROTEIN **14.1 g**	CARBOHYDRATE **25.3 g**	FAT **15.6 g**

²/₃ cup (100 g) quinoa (I use a red and white mixture)

Salt and freshly ground black pepper

1 Pink Lady apple, cored and sliced

1 pear, cored and sliced

1 ripe avocado, peeled, pitted, sliced, and tossed in a little lemon juice

4 ounces (100 g) reduced-fat hard cheese, cut into chunks

¼ cup (25 g) whole almonds

A few pomegranate seeds

1. Rinse the quinoa in a strainer, place in a pan, and cover with 1⅓ cups (315 ml) of cold water. Add a pinch of salt, bring to a boil, lower the heat, and cook gently for 10 to 15 minutes, until tender. Drain and rinse in cold water to cool quickly, then drain again. Season with salt and pepper, if desired.

2. Divide the quinoa among 4 serving bowls and arrange the apple, pear, and avocado slices on top with the cheese and almonds.

3. Sprinkle with the pomegranate seeds to serve.

Asian Salmon Burgers

I adore fish cakes, but some can be very disappointing, if lacking in fish or flavor. The best way to overcome this is to make your own, and I often do so without the help of potato or bread crumbs in the mix. These are a firm favorite—salmon ones flavored with scallions, ginger, lime, cilantro, and fish sauce. All they require is a little salad on the side to make a great light meal.

	SERVES 4		
PER PORTION:	CALORIES **200**	PROTEIN **21.5 g**	CARBOHYDRATE **1.2 g**	FAT **11.9 g**

14 ounces (400 g) salmon fillets, skinned and cut into chunks

5 scallions, roughly chopped

2 teaspoons grated peeled fresh ginger

Small bunch cilantro

Grated zest of 1 lime

1 teaspoon fish sauce

Salt and freshly ground black pepper

Low-fat cooking spray

Lime wedges and crisp salad, to serve

1. Place about one-third of the salmon into a food processor with the scallions, ginger, cilantro, lime zest, fish sauce, and salt and pepper. Blend until roughly combined, but don't let it become a smooth paste. Add the remaining salmon and pulse a few times to mix. You should still be able to see some chunks of fish. Chill for about 30 minutes or until firm enough to handle.

2. With wet hands, divide and shape the fish mixture into 4 burgers, and chill again to firm, if time allows. Preheat the oven to 400°F (200°C).

3. Generously spray a large frying pan with low-fat cooking spray. Heat, add the burgers, and cook over medium heat for 2 minutes on each side, until golden. Transfer to a nonstick baking sheet. Bake for 8 minutes, or until cooked through.

4. Serve hot, with lime wedges for squeezing over, and a crisp side salad.

Zesty Lime Shrimp with Avocado

This simple dish of shrimp and avocado dressed with a lime and cilantro mixture makes a wonderful light lunch dish. Serve with a little bread, if you can tolerate it, for a more substantial meal.

○ ○ ●   SERVES **4**

PER PORTION:	CALORIES **185**	PROTEIN **21.7 g**	CARBOHYDRATE **3.8 g**	FAT **9.5 g**

1 pound (450 g) cooked peeled and deveined shrimp

1 tomato, chopped

1 avocado, peeled, pitted, chopped, and tossed in a little lemon or lime juice

1 small jalapeño pepper, seeded and chopped

¼ red onion, finely chopped

Grated zest of 1 lime

Juice of 2 limes

1 teaspoon olive oil

1 tablespoon chopped fresh cilantro

Salt and freshly ground black pepper

Lime wedges, to serve (optional)

1. Mix the shrimp with the tomato, avocado, jalapeño, and red onion in a bowl.
2. Mix the lime zest with the lime juice, oil, cilantro, and salt and pepper, and pour over the shrimp mixture. Toss to mix well.
3. Serve with lime wedges for squeezing over, if desired.

Ham, Scallion, and Feta Frittata

WLS PORTION: ½–1

Sandwiches, pies, and chips were my pre-op choice of lunch box, picnic, or buffet table fare, but these days, I'm more choosy! One of my staples for such occasions is a frittata—a wedge served on a bed of mixed greens proves perfect for dining events and can be made quickly and easily with leftovers as well as newly purchased food items. This one is made with new potatoes and a little feta, eggs. and a thick slice of carved ham. With some chopped fresh mint from the garden, you have the makings of a fine feast. But you could make it with almost any leftovers. It's delicious hot, warm, or cold.

			SERVES **4**		
PER PORTION:	CALORIES **177**	PROTEIN **14.6 g**	CARBOHYDRATE **9.6 g**	FAT **8.9 g**

7 ounces (200 g) new potatoes

6 scallions, trimmed

Low-fat cooking oil or spray

1 thick slice carved ham or about 3 ounces (75 g) ham slices, roughly torn

4 eggs, beaten

Generous ½ cup (60 g) crumbled reduced-fat feta cheese

6 fresh mint leaves, chopped

Salt and freshly ground black pepper

1. Chop the potatoes into bite-size chunks and parcook in boiling water for 5 to 7 minutes, until almost tender. Add the scallions for the last 1 minute of the cooking time, then drain well.

2. Generously spray a medium nonstick frying or sauté pan with low-fat cooking spray and heat over medium heat. Add the potatoes, scallions, and ham, and heat through for 1 minute.

3. Add the eggs and stir a few times to coat and incorporate everything together. Sprinkle over the feta and mint, and season with salt and pepper. Allow to cook gently for about 8 to 10 minutes, or until almost cooked through. Meanwhile, heat the broiler.

4. Transfer the pan to the broiler and cook until the frittata is golden on top and cooked through—about 3 to 5 minutes.

5. Serve hot or warm and cut into wedges, or allow to cool and then slice to serve.

Creamy Tuna Salad

Tuna salad is a firm favorite in my lunch box, but I used to make it with a combination of mayo and yogurt to make a creamy soft mixture. This is an alternative, where no mayo is required at all. The creaminess comes from the avocado used to bind the ingredients together. This means that the fat stats might be a bit higher, but they're good fats! I've used canned albacore tuna in water but you can use fresh cooked tuna instead. It makes a great buffet dish or topping for a baked potato, too.

			SERVES **4** (as a side dish)/**2** (as a main course salad)		
PER PORTION:	CALORIES **160/320**	PROTEIN **14 g/28 g**	CARBOHYDRATE **3.5 g/7 g**		FAT **10.1 g/20.2 g**

1 large ripe avocado, peeled and pitted

2 tablespoons lemon or lime juice

Salt and freshly ground black pepper

Half a 14-ounce (400 g) can albacore tuna in water, drained and flaked

1 small red onion, thinly sliced

½ small cucumber, thinly sliced

3 tablespoons chopped cilantro, chives, or parsley

1. Mash half the avocado with a fork until almost smooth. Stir in the lemon or lime juice and salt and pepper. Slice or chop the remaining avocado into bite-size chunks.
2. Mix the tuna in a bowl with the red onion, cucumber, and cilantro or other herbs.
3. Add the prepared avocado "cream" and avocado chunks or slices, and fold gently together to mix. Cover and chill until ready to serve.

NOTE: If you are at the early onset of the Soft Food (Yellow) stage, feel free to purée or fork-mash the entire recipe to a suitable texture and consistency.

Pear Necessities Blue Cheese Salad

WLS PORTION: ½–1

This is a lovely salad to eat when pears are at their best—firm but tender and ripe—and ideal with crispy salad greens and nuggets of blue cheese. The lemony dressing is spiked with poppy seeds for visual interest and provides just enough sharpness to balance the sweetness of the pears.

○ ○ ●	SERVES 2	Ⓥ

PER PORTION:	CALORIES **300**	PROTEIN **10.1 g**	CARBOHYDRATE **18.7 g**	FAT **20.3 g**

7 ounces (200 g) crispy salad greens (radicchio and frisée with lettuce and watercress makes a good mix)

2 ripe pears, quartered, cored, and sliced

3 ounces (75 g) blue cheese, crumbled

For the Dressing

Grated zest and juice of ½ lemon

1 tablespoon oil

2 teaspoons poppy seeds

Small pinch of sugar or sweetener

Salt and freshly ground black pepper

1. Divide the salad greens between 2 plates or place in a salad bowl. Top with the sliced pear and crumbled blue cheese.
2. **To make the dressing,** whisk the lemon zest, lemon juice, oil, poppy seeds, sugar or sweetener, and salt and pepper.
3. Drizzle the dressing over the salad, toss to mix, and serve immediately.

Quinoa, Nectarine, and Sizzled Halloumi Salad

WLS PORTION: ½

Nectarines (or peaches, if you prefer) taste amazingly good with halloumi cheese, and the quinoa and almonds add yet more bite and texture to this salad. Choose almost any low-fat or fat-free dressing that you like, but a mustard one works particularly well.

○ ○ ●	SERVES 4	Ⓥ

PER PORTION:	CALORIES 254	PROTEIN 12.2 g	CARBOHYDRATE 23.2 g	FAT 12.4 g

½ cup (85 g) quinoa

1 vegetable bouillon cube

2 nectarines, pitted and sliced

Large handful of spinach, watercress, and/or arugula

¼ cup (25 g) whole almonds, toasted

4 ounces (125 g) halloumi cheese, sliced

2 tablespoons pomegranate seeds

3 tablespoons low-fat or fat-free dressing

1. Rinse the quinoa in a strainer, then cook in simmering water with the bouillon cube for 15 minutes, or until tender. Drain well and let cool slightly.
2. Mix the warm quinoa with the nectarines and spinach and watercress. Divide among 4 serving plates and scatter the almonds on top.
3. Heat a large nonstick frying pan and fry the slices of halloumi cheese for 1 to 2 minutes on each side, until golden. Divide among the salads.
4. Sprinkle with the pomegranate seeds and drizzle with the dressing to serve.

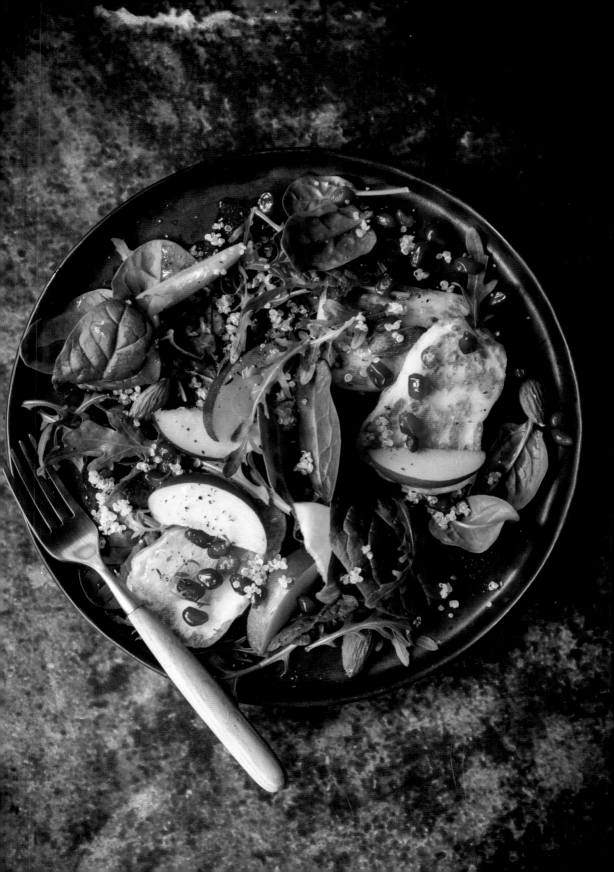

Strawberry, Bean, and Herb Salad

WLS
PORTION:
½

This is a deceptively simple salad made with beans, strawberries, red onion, and herbs. It tastes fabulous on its own but exceptional with some peppered smoked mackerel or salmon. You can of course make the salad stretch further by adding some flaked fish, deli meats, roast poultry, cheese, or vegetarian options, and boost the protein, too. It will keep for one to two days in the fridge. Eat at home for a light lunch or pack up and take on a picnic.

		SERVES 2		Ⓥ
PER PORTION:	CALORIES **145**	PROTEIN **9 g**	CARBOHYDRATE **25.4 g**	FAT **0.6 g**

One 14-ounce (400 g) can cannellini beans (or other white beans), drained and rinsed

½ small red onion, thinly sliced

10 strawberries, hulled and sliced

2 tablespoons chopped fresh mint

1 tablespoon snipped chives

¼ cup (60 ml) low-fat or fat-free French-style dressing

Salt and freshly ground black pepper

1. Place the beans in a bowl with the red onion, strawberries, mint, and chives, and mix gently.
2. Add the dressing with salt and pepper to taste. Cover and chill until ready to serve.

Pink Lady Apple Chicken Salad
with Butternut Bites

WLS
PORTION:
½

This salad checks all the boxes for a healthy bariatric meal—high protein and good complex carbs plus great flavor and crunch. Replace the butternut squash with sweet potato if you prefer, but increase the cooking time slightly.

○ ○ ●	SERVES 2		
PER PORTION: CALORIES **365**	PROTEIN **33.2 g**	CARBOHYDRATE **25.3 g**	FAT **14.6 g**

11 ounces (300 g) butternut squash, peeled, seeded, and cut into bite-size chunks

Low-fat cooking spray

Pinch of cumin seeds or crushed red pepper flakes (optional)

¼ cup (25 g) whole hazelnuts

3 ounces (80 g) spinach, watercress, and arugula salad

1 Pink Lady apple, cored and sliced

8 ounces (225 g) skinless, boneless roast chicken, torn into pieces

¼ cup plus 2 tablespoons (90 ml) fat-free vinaigrette

1 teaspoon Dijon mustard

1. Preheat the oven to 400°F (200°C). Put the butternut squash in a roasting pan and spray generously with low-fat cooking spray. Roast for 20 minutes.

2. Turn the chunks over, sprinkle with cumin seeds or crushed red pepper flakes, if using, and add the hazelnuts. Roast for 4 to 5 more minutes.

3. Divide the salad greens between 2 serving plates. Top with the apple and cooked chicken. Scatter over the cooked butternut squash with hazelnuts.

4. Mix the dressing with the mustard and drizzle over the salads to serve.

Beet and Parsnip Fritters with Horseradish Yogurt Drizzle

Root vegetables add sweetness and flavor to a dish that can delight the jaded bariatric palate. Make them into fritters and drizzle with a mouth-tingling sauce, and you have a great fresh and punchy light meal. A simple arugula salad makes a good accompaniment.

○ ○ ●		SERVES **4**		**V**
PER PORTION:	CALORIES **165**	PROTEIN **9.3 g**	CARBOHYDRATE **21.7 g**	FAT **4.4 g**

Low-fat cooking spray

1 onion, chopped

2 garlic cloves, crushed

2 parsnips (about 7 ounces/200 g), peeled and coarsely grated

2 carrots, peeled and coarsely grated

2 beets (about 11 ounces/300 g), peeled and coarsely grated

2 eggs, beaten

1 small bunch fresh dill, chopped

2 teaspoons chopped fresh mint

Salt and freshly ground black pepper

1 cup (175 g) fat-free plain or coconut yogurt

1½ teaspoons prepared horseradish

1. Generously spray a small skillet with low-fat cooking spray. Heat, add the onion and garlic, and cook until softened, about 5 minutes. Set aside.
2. Mix the parsnips with the carrot and beets, then squeeze with hands or in a paper towel to remove as much liquid as possible.
3. Add the eggs, half of the dill, the mint, the cooked onion and garlic, and salt and pepper, and mix well.
4. Generously spray a large frying pan with low-fat cooking spray. Heat over medium heat, then add heaping spoonfuls of the mixture to the pan to make patty shapes about 2½ inches (6 cm) in diameter. You will have to cook in 2 to 3 batches, and the mixture will make about 12 fritters. Cook for 3 to 4 minutes on each side, turning very gently with a spatula. It may be necessary to spray the pan again between batches. Keep warm.
5. Meanwhile, mix the remaining dill with the yogurt and horseradish.
6. Serve the fritters warm with the sauce drizzled over.

Venison with Sprout and Apple Slaw

Venison is one of the leanest meats around and packs a great protein punch. I find it needs a bit of marinating to get some additional flavor before cooking—and I like it cooked rare. It makes a great light lunch for a bariatric if served with a crunchy slaw. This one uses finely shredded sprouts (try it if you are skeptical, and see how good it is), apple and pomegranate seeds in a crème fraîche dressing. Wonderfully festive and a great light meal or starter dish.

○ ○ ●		SERVES **4**		
PER PORTION:	CALORIES **225**	PROTEIN **25.7 g**	CARBOHYDRATE **9.3 g**	FAT **9 g**

For the Venison
2 tablespoons olive oil
½ teaspoon balsamic vinegar
1 tablespoon Worcestershire sauce
1 teaspoon chopped fresh rosemary
2 juniper berries, crushed
Salt and freshly ground black pepper
14 ounces (400 g) boneless venison loin

For the Slaw
8 ounces (225 g) Brussels sprouts, finely shredded
Grated zest and juice of ½ orange
1 green apple, cored and grated
¼ cup (15 g) chopped fresh parsley
3 tablespoons pomegranate seeds
3 tablespoons reduced-fat crème fraîche
½–1 teaspoon prepared horseradish

1. Mix the oil with the vinegar, Worcestershire sauce, rosemary, juniper berries, and salt and pepper to make the marinade. Marinate the venison in the refrigerator for at least 2 hours (or ideally overnight).
2. Preheat the oven to 400°F (200°C).
3. Heat a cast-iron skillet until very hot. Add the venison and cook for 2 to 3 minutes, until well-browned and caramelized on the underside. Turn and cook for 2 more minutes, so that it is browned and sealed on all sides.
4. Place on a baking sheet and cook in the oven for 5 to 6 minutes, depending upon how rare you like your venison cooked. Remove from the oven and let stand for 5 minutes, then slice.
5. **To make the slaw,** meanwhile, mix the Brussels sprouts with the orange zest, orange juice, apple, parsley, pomegranate seeds, and salt and pepper. Mix the crème fraîche with the horseradish and fold into the slaw mixture to coat.
6. Serve the sliced venison with the slaw on the side.

Satay Chicken Skewers

These chicken skewers pair wonderfully with my Simple Shallot Satay Sauce (page 206). I like to prepare and cook mine in a ridged grill pan, but you can of course cook them on the barbecue or under the broiler, too. They are fabulous served hot, warm, or cold, and make a great addition to a packed lunch box as well as a main meal choice. I don't believe you need to add much more than a mixed side salad to make a great WLS meal.

○ ○ ●		SERVES **4**		
PER PORTION:	CALORIES **185**	PROTEIN **36.6 g**	CARBOHYDRATE **0.8 g**	FAT **3.9 g**

1 teaspoon olive oil

Juice of 1 lime

½ teaspoon crushed red pepper flakes

2 teaspoons soy sauce

Salt and freshly ground black pepper

3 boneless, skinless chicken breasts (about 6 ounces/175 g each), cut into long, thin strips or cubes

1. Soak 16 bamboo or wooden skewers in water for 15 minutes.
2. Mix the oil with the lime juice, crushed red pepper flakes, soy sauce, and salt and pepper. Add the chicken strips or cubes and toss well to coat. Cover and let marinate for at least 30 minutes or overnight in the fridge.
3. To cook, thread the chicken onto the soaked skewers. If you are using a grill pan, heat it over medium heat and cook the chicken skewers for 3 to 4 minutes on each side, or until browned and cooked through. Barbecue over medium-hot coals, or broil under medium–high heat, for about 3 minutes each side, turning frequently.
4. Serve with Simple Shallot Satay Sauce (page 206) and lime wedges for squeezing over.

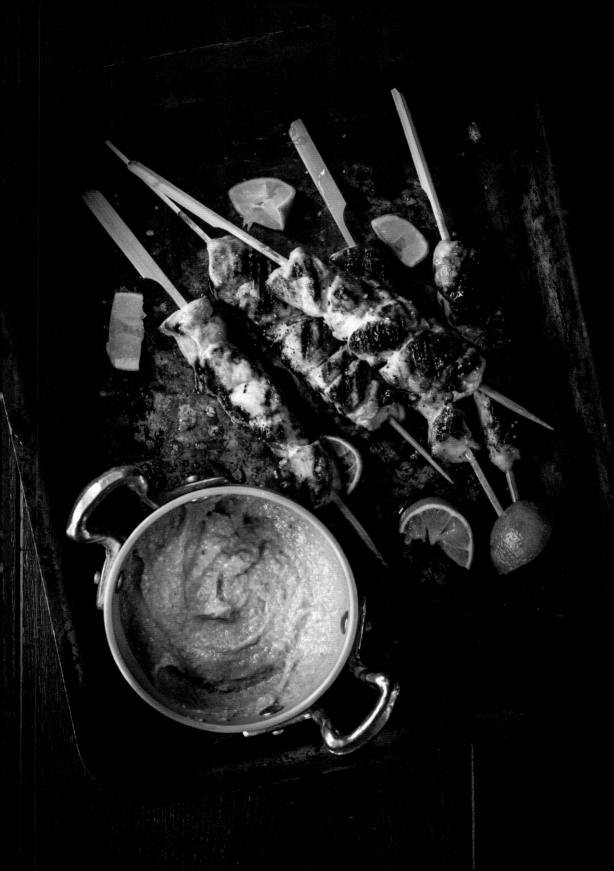

Main Meals

Pacific Cod with Pepper Stir-Fry

Here's a very simple fish recipe that is perfect for main meal eating. It is endlessly versatile if you use different vegetables that are suitable for stir-frying. Next time why not try sliced green beans, sugar snap peas, sliced carrot, red onion, zucchini, and broccoli florets?

○ ○ ● | SERVES **4**

PER PORTION:	CALORIES **227**	PROTEIN **33.3 g**	CARBOHYDRATE **13.9 g**	FAT **3.9 g**

Low-fat cooking spray

Four 6-ounce (175 g) skinless cod fillets

Finely grated zest and juice of 1 lime

6 scallions, sliced

2 red bell peppers, cored, seeded, and thinly sliced

2 yellow bell peppers, cored, seeded, and thinly sliced

4 ounces (125 g) green beans, halved

About 8 canned baby corn, halved if large

8 ounces (225 g) bean sprouts

Soy sauce

Freshly ground black pepper

1. Preheat the broiler. Cover the broiler pan-rack with foil and spray with low-fat cooking spray. Arrange the cod fillets on top. Sprinkle with the lime zest, lime juice, and a few slices of the scallions. Broil for 6 to 8 minutes, until the flesh is opaque and will flake easily.

2. Meanwhile, liberally spray a large frying pan or wok with low-fat cooking spray. Heat, add the bell peppers, remaining scallions, green beans, and baby corn. Stir-fry for 3 to 4 minutes. Add the bean sprouts and stir-fry for 1 to 2 more minutes.

3. Divide the stir-fry among 4 serving plates and top each one with a cod fillet. Season to taste with soy sauce and freshly ground black pepper to serve.

One-Pan Wonder Thai Sea Bass

When you have one eye on the clock and a meal to make, "one-pan wonder" recipes come to the fore. Meat, fish, poultry, and vegetables in imaginative combinations all cooked together in one pan work well. This fish has been given the Thai treatment. I have used asparagus, bok choy, and scallions as my vegetable base, but you can use whatever is in season or whatever you have on hand (just remember your cooking times might change). The key seasonings of ginger, garlic, chile, fish sauce, soy sauce, and lime or lemon juice are, however, essential, but throw in some chopped cilantro if you have some, too. I have used oil for this dish so that it produces a wonderful juice for serving with the sea bass, but it does raise the fat profile. If you're an avid fat-checker, then spray instead with low-fat cooking spray and the fat will be minimal.

○ ○ ● | SERVES 2

PER PORTION:	CALORIES 355	PROTEIN 24.2 g	CARBOHYDRATE 6.1 g	FAT 26.4 g

4 ounces (100 g) asparagus spears, trimmed

7 ounces (200 g, about 2 medium) bok choy, quartered

2 scallions, chopped

2 garlic cloves, crushed

1 mild red chile, seeded and sliced

¼ cup (100 g) grated peeled fresh ginger

3 tablespoons oil (I use sesame oil)

1 tablespoon fish sauce (Nam Pla)

1 tablespoon soy sauce

Grated zest and juice of 1 lime or 1 small lemon

2 sea bass fillets (about 7 ounces/190 g)

2 tablespoons chopped fresh cilantro (optional)

1. Preheat the oven to 400°F (200°C).
2. Place the asparagus, bok choy, and scallions in a medium roasting pan.
3. Mix the garlic with the chile, ginger, oil, fish sauce, soy sauce, and lime or lemon zest and juice in a bowl. Add half of the mixture to the vegetables and toss well to coat. Roast for 5 minutes.
4. Remove from the oven and top with the sea bass fillets. Return to the oven and cook for 8 minutes, or until the sea bass is cooked—it will flake easily when tested with the tip of a knife, and the flesh should look opaque.
5. Spoon the remaining oil mixture over the fish to serve, sprinkled with chopped cilantro, if desired.
6. Serve with jasmine rice, noodles, potatoes, or without any additions, as preferred.

Simple Fish Stew

WLS PORTION:
½–¾

Here's a speedy and simple fish stew that is simply loaded with protein. It makes a great nourishing bowlful for a bariatric, and any leftovers can be stored in the refrigerator for two to three days for another meal. Non-WLS diners may appreciate a little crusty bread on the side to mop up all the juices. This quantity will serve four but the portion size isn't huge—add more lima beans to stretch if you are catering for hearty appetites.

			SERVES **4**	
PER PORTION:	CALORIES **245**	PROTEIN **27.6 g**	CARBOHYDRATE **20.8 g**	FAT **3.4 g**

Low-fat cooking spray

1 small onion, sliced

2 garlic cloves, crushed

Pinch of crushed red pepper flakes

1 teaspoon smoked paprika

One 14-ounce (400 g) can diced tomatoes

3¼ cups (750 ml) vegetable stock

One 14-ounce (400 g) can lima beans, drained and rinsed

11 ounces (300 g) white fish fillets, cut into bite-size chunks

1 cup (150 g) peeled and deveined shrimp

Salt and freshly ground black pepper

Lemon wedges and chopped fresh parsley, to garnish

1. Generously spray a large pan with low-fat cooking spray. Heat, add the onion and garlic, and cook gently for about 8 minutes, until softened.
2. Stir in the crushed red pepper flakes and paprika, mixing well. Add the tomatoes and stock and bring to a boil. Simmer gently for 10 minutes.
3. Reduce the heat, add the beans and fish, and simmer until the fish is almost cooked through, about 4 minutes.
4. Add the shrimp and cook until they turn pink and opaque.
5. Season with salt and pepper, ladle into bowls to serve, and garnish with lemon wedges for squeezing over the stew and chopped parsley.

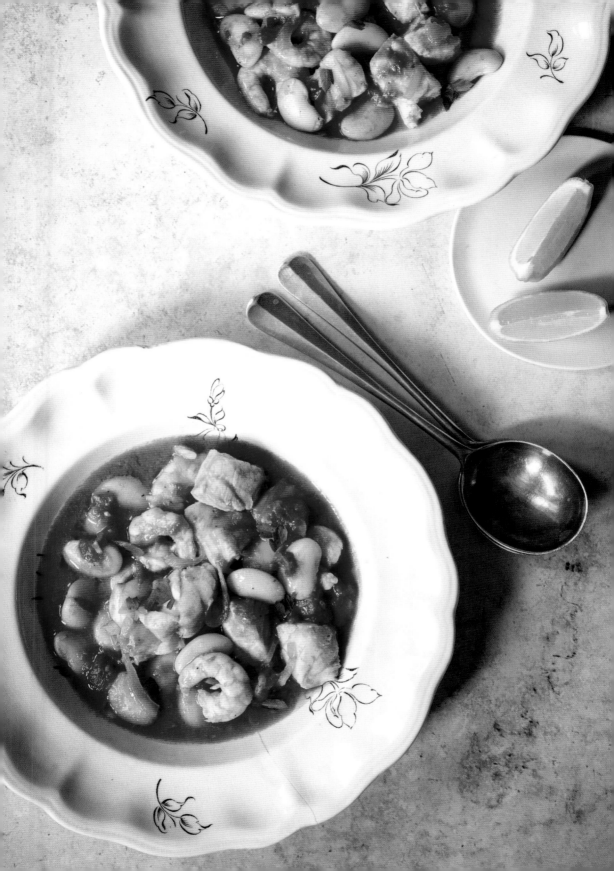

Salmon, Asparagus, and Squash Rice Bowl

This is just the kind of food I like—simple to prepare and on the table in no time but looks like you have been laboring for hours. This recipe serves two but can easily be doubled or tripled, and the rice is somewhat optional—I often do without, but bigger eaters find it extends the meal.

○ ○ ● | SERVES **2**

PER PORTION:	CALORIES **465**	PROTEIN **35.5 g**	CARBOHYDRATE **47.6 g**	FAT **14.8 g**

1 pound (500 g) butternut squash, peeled, seeded, and chopped into bite-size pieces

Low-fat cooking spray

2 teaspoons cumin seeds

Pinch of crushed red pepper flakes

Salt and freshly ground black pepper

2 teaspoons grated peeled fresh ginger

2 salmon fillets (about 8 ounces/250 g)

2 teaspoons honey (optional)

1 bunch asparagus spears, trimmed

7 ounces (200 g) warm, cooked long-grain brown rice

1 tablespoon peanuts, chopped

Cilantro sprigs and lemon wedges, to garnish

1. Preheat the oven to 425°F (220°C).
2. Generously spray the squash with low-fat cooking spray and toss with the cumin seeds, crushed red pepper flakes, and salt and pepper. Place on a large baking sheet and roast for 25 minutes.
3. Meanwhile, rub the ginger over the salmon and drizzle with the honey, if using. Season to taste with salt and pepper.
4. Add the asparagus and salmon to the pan with the squash after 25 minutes, and roast for an additional 10 minutes.
5. To serve, put the squash, asparagus, and rice in 2 serving bowls and top each with a cooked salmon fillet. Sprinkle with the peanuts and garnish with cilantro and lemon wedges to squeeze over before serving.

Honey-Mustard Roast Salmon

WLS
PORTION:
½

The simplicity of this dish belies its finished look and taste. Salmon fillets (great for protein) are coated with mustard flavored with honey, garlic, paprika, lemon juice, and chives, and baked until nicely browned. You can sprinkle with some sesame seeds for the last five minutes of roasting, if desired. I like to serve with steamed vegetables and a little mashed potato.

○ ○ ● | SERVES **2**

PER PORTION:	CALORIES **220**	PROTEIN **22.3 g**	CARBOHYDRATE **2.3 g**	FAT **13.5 g**

Low-fat cooking spray

2 salmon fillets, about 4 ounces (100 g) each

2 tablespoons honey-mustard

2 garlic cloves, crushed

Juice of ½ lemon

½ teaspoon smoked paprika

1 tablespoon snipped fresh chives

Salt and freshly ground black pepper

1. Preheat the oven to 400°F (200°C).

2. Spray a rimmed baking sheet with low-fat cooking spray. Place the salmon on the baking sheet. Mix the mustard with the garlic, lemon juice, paprika, chives, and salt and pepper. Brush or spoon over the salmon.

3. Roast for 15 to 20 minutes (depending upon thickness), until cooked through and browned. Serve hot.

Hoisin-Glazed Shrimp

Shrimp are fabulously good for protein, but they often need a bit of a lift with seasoning to tantalize the taste buds. I find cooking with hoisin sauce gives a sweet-savory flavor that checks the boxes on all counts. Choose a sauce that is as low in sugar as possible and then add a few strips of green beans, thin asparagus spears, or scallions for crunch. I like to serve with just a few vermicelli noodles but always eat the shrimp first.

○ ○ ● | SERVES **2**

PER PORTION (with noodles):	CALORIES **150**	PROTEIN **21 g**	CARBOHYDRATE **10.8 g**	FAT **2.6 g**

8 ounces (250 g) large peeled and deveined shrimp

¼ cup hoisin sauce

1 teaspoon sesame oil or low-fat cooking spray

2 shallots, chopped

2 teaspoons grated peeled fresh ginger

1 large garlic clove, crushed

About 4 ounces (100 g) trimmed thin French beans, thin asparagus spears, or julienned zucchini

Salt and freshly ground black pepper

½ teaspoon Malay spice mix (optional)

3 tablespoons soy sauce

2 scallions, chopped, or 2 tablespoons chopped cilantro

Vermicelli noodles, to serve (optional)

1 teaspoon toasted sesame seeds or 1 tablespoon crushed peanuts, to sprinkle

1. Place the shrimp in a bowl with the hoisin sauce and mix well.
2. Heat the oil in a pan or wok (or generously spray a pan with low-fat cooking spray and heat). Add the shallots, ginger, garlic, and prepared vegetables, and stir-fry for about 3 minutes, until tender-crisp. Remove with a slotted spoon and reserve.
3. Add the shrimp, reserving any hoisin sauce, and cook for about 4 minutes, turning occasionally, until pink and opaque.
4. Return the vegetable mixture to the pan with the reserved hoisin sauce and salt and pepper. Add the Malay spice, if using, and soy sauce, mixing well. Cook for 1 minute.
5. Add the scallions or cilantro and toss well to serve.
6. Serve plain or with noodles, if desired, and sprinkle with sesame seeds or crushed peanuts.

Creamy White Chicken Chili

White chicken chili is a version of chili made with chicken instead of beef, using white beans instead of red or black, and thickened with a white sauce rather than a red one. It often has more chiles than my version here, but spiciness and hotness are not good for WLS patients, so I have kept it quite low (add more if you like). I like to serve this with a little cauliflower rice, but it's just fine on its own or spooned over a baked potato. This recipe also uses a canned soup as a shortcut for the base—there are many low-fat and low-sugar versions to choose from—check the labels to be sure.

SERVES **4**

PER PORTION:	CALORIES **375**	PROTEIN **50.3 g**	CARBOHYDRATE **32 g**	FAT **4.5 g**

Low-fat cooking spray

1 pound (450 g) skinless and boneless chicken breast or thigh meat, cut into strips

1 onion, chopped

1½ teaspoons ground cumin

Two 14-ounce (400 g) cans low-fat and low-sugar chicken soup or broth

Two 14-ounce (400 g) cans white beans (such as cannellini), drained and rinsed

4 ounces (100 g) canned chiles, chopped

1 cup (100 g) grated low-fat hard cheese

Salt and freshly ground black pepper

1. Spray a large nonstick pan with low-fat cooking spray. Heat, add the chicken and onion and cook until the chicken is no longer pink, but do not allow to brown.
2. Add the cumin and cook for 1 minute.
3. Add the soup or broth, beans, and chiles, mixing well. Bring to a boil, lower the heat to a simmer, cover, and cook for about 10 to 15 minutes, until the chicken is tender and the flavors have developed.
4. Just before serving, stir in the cheese until melted, and season to taste with salt and pepper. Serve hot.

   NOTE: If you are at the early onset of the Soft Food (Yellow) stage, then feel free to purée or fork-mash the entire recipe to a suitable texture and consistency.

One-Pan Roasted Chicken with Mediterranean Vegetables

WLS PORTION: ½

Roast chicken is one of the staples of the WLS dietary regimen, but it has its problems. First, it can be tough and indigestible unless cooked super-tender. Second, a whole bird takes quite some time to cook, and when you have a meal to cook and little time, it can be off-limits. Third, it needs accompaniments, which also takes time and effort to prepare. The solution? A one-pan chicken thigh dish (no extras needed) that cooks succulent and tender, and can be on the table comfortably in under an hour. As a bonus, the leftovers (should there be any) can be chilled and reheated with confidence, or frozen for eating on a time-strapped day.

○ ○ ● | SERVES **4**

PER PORTION (with skin-on chicken):	CALORIES **403**	PROTEIN **54.7 g**	CARBOHYDRATE **13.6 g**	FAT **15.1 g**

1 red onion, cut into wedges

1 zucchini, cut into bite-size pieces

1 yellow bell pepper, cored, seeded, and cut into chunks

1 red bell pepper, cored, seeded, and cut into chunks

1 eggplant, cut into chunks

Low-fat cooking spray

8 chicken thighs (skinned, if desired)

1 tablespoon chopped fresh thyme

3 tablespoons soy sauce

¾ cup (200 ml) chicken stock

¼ cup (60 ml) reduced-fat, low-sugar tomato pasta sauce or passata (crushed tomatoes)

1. Preheat the oven to 350°F (180°C).
2. Place the onion, zucchini, bell peppers, and eggplant in a large nonstick roasting pan. Liberally spray with low-fat cooking spray to coat on all sides.
3. Tuck the chicken thighs among the vegetables, and sprinkle with the thyme. Roast for 30 minutes, turning occasionally so that they cook evenly.
4. Mix the soy sauce with the chicken stock and pasta sauce or passata, and pour into the pan over the vegetables and around the chicken thighs.
5. Return to the oven for a further 15 to 20 minutes, or until the chicken is cooked through and the vegetables are tender.

VARIATION **One-Pan Roasted Chicken with Winter Vegetables:** For those who want a winter mix (and are not overly concerned about carbs) use a selection of potato (white or sweet) and root vegetables, such as parsnips, carrots, turnips, or celeriac. Parboil even-size chunks of them for about 5 minutes, then drain well so that they cook in the same time as the chicken.

Creamy Pepper Chicken Skillet

The beauty of chicken breast fillets or tenders is that not only do they have great protein but they also can be cooked quickly and are super gentle on the bariatric pouch. Here they are combined with bell peppers and a light cream cheese for a dish that's hard to beat. Serve with a little rice, pasta, or vegetables, if desired.

○ ○ ● | SERVES **4**

PER PORTION:	CALORIES **205**	PROTEIN **34.6 g**	CARBOHYDRATE **10.9 g**	FAT **3 g**

Low-fat cooking spray

1 onion, sliced

4 bell peppers (red, green, yellow, or orange, or a mixture), cored, seeded, and thinly sliced

1 pound (450 g) skinless and boneless chicken breasts, or chicken tenders, cut into strips

¼ cup (50 g) light cream cheese (with herbs, if desired)

Salt and freshly ground black pepper

1. Generously spray a nonstick pan or skillet with low-fat cooking spray. Heat, add the onion and bell peppers, and cook for 5 to 7 minutes, until softened, stirring occasionally. Remove from the pan and keep warm.

2. Add the chicken and a little extra spray, if necessary, and cook until no longer pink, about 3 to 4 minutes each side.

3. Return the pepper mixture to the pan and mix well. Add the cream cheese and season with salt and pepper, and cook for 1 to 2 minutes, or until the cheese has melted and the sauce is creamy.

4. Serve hot with rice, pasta, or vegetables of your choice.

Barbecue Chicken

Here is a recipe that I return to time and time again because it is so popular and suits just about everyone, young and old, fussy and adventurous, WLS patient and not. Unlike many other marinated chicken dishes, this doesn't need any substantial prep-time for a tasty result. It's amazingly good as an impromptu dish when the sun makes a welcome appearance.

○ ○ ● | SERVES **4**

PER PORTION:	CALORIES **275**	PROTEIN **37.1 g**	CARBOHYDRATE **7.2 g**	FAT **10.4 g**

2 teaspoons chopped peeled fresh ginger

½ cup (150 ml) low-sugar ketchup

3 tablespoons Worcestershire sauce

Salt and freshly ground black pepper

1½ pounds (750 g) skinless bone-in chicken thighs

Sprout and Apple Slaw (page 149), to serve (optional)

1. In a large bowl, mix the ginger with the ketchup, Worcestershire sauce, and season with salt and pepper.
2. Slash the top side of the chicken thighs with a knife to make deep cuts, then add to the bowl and mix until evenly coated, making sure the marinade goes into the slashes. Let stand for 10 minutes or longer.
3. Broil or barbecue over medium heat for about 25 minutes, turning once or twice, until nicely browned and cooked through without any pink meat.
4. Serve hot with the slaw, if desired.

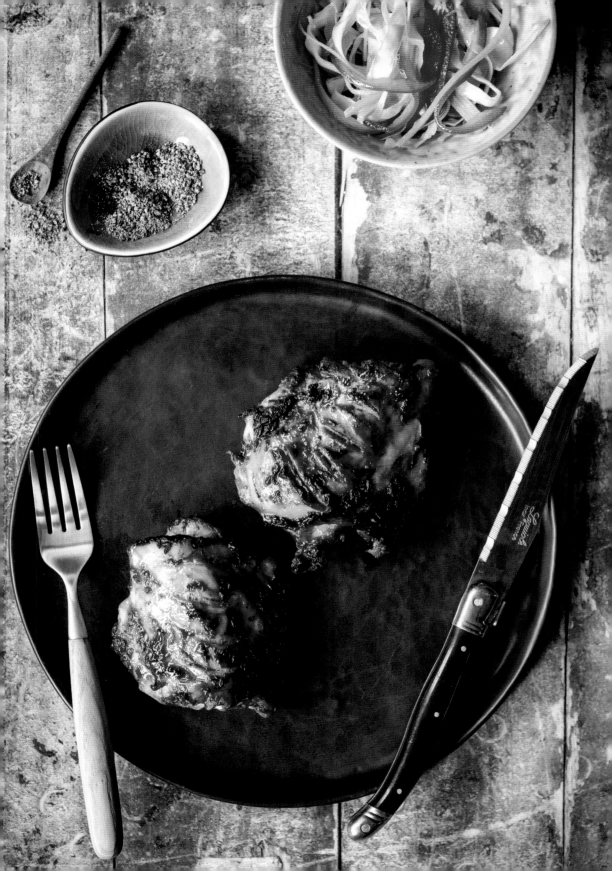

Stuffed Mushrooms, Fajita-Style

WLS
PORTION:
1

I already substitute portobello mushrooms for the bun in burger recipes, and I also use them as bases for holding other savory ingredients that can be baked for an easy dinner. This one features classic fajita-style ingredients but stays low-carb without the tortillas.

		MAKES 6	

PER PORTION:	CALORIES 115	PROTEIN 19 g	CARBOHYDRATE 6.3 g	FAT 1.5 g

6 large portobello mushrooms

Low-fat cooking spray

1 onion, sliced

1 green bell pepper, cored, seeded, and sliced

4 tomatoes, chopped

½ teaspoon chili powder

½ teaspoon ground cumin

½ teaspoon paprika

1½ cups (300 g) diced cooked chicken

Salt and freshly ground black pepper

½ cup (50 g) grated low-fat hard cheese

1. Preheat the oven to 350°F (180°C).
2. Clean the mushrooms, then spray liberally on all sides with low-fat cooking spray. Place on a baking sheet and bake for 10 minutes.
3. Meanwhile, liberally spray a pan with low-fat cooking spray. Heat, add the onion and bell pepper, and cook until softened, about 5 to 7 minutes.
4. Add the tomatoes, chili powder, cumin, paprika, chicken, and salt and pepper, mixing well. Cook for 5 minutes.
5. Fill the mushroom caps with the chicken mixture and top with the cheese. Bake for 10 to 15 minutes, or until the cheese is melted and golden. Serve hot.

Ginger and Lemon Chicken Stir-Fry

WLS PORTION: ½

Oh, how we ache for something with crunch soon after surgery, and a stir-fry looks so beguiling. It can certainly come back onto the menu eventually, but initially, you may have to make sure that you cook the ingredients on the tender side and then raise the heat and cook them faster to a crisper result as you proceed further along the WLS journey. You will have fun mixing and matching ingredients. My only word of caution is to consider carefully your choice of stir-fry sauce or marinade. Some have huge amounts of sugar, salt, and believe it or not, fat or oil in them, so check the ingredients or, better still, make your own. The simplest is to use equal quantities of soy sauce and Worcestershire sauce and use this as a marinade prior to cooking.

		SERVES 2		
PER PORTION:	CALORIES **170**	PROTEIN **33 g**	CARBOHYDRATE **5.4 g**	FAT **1.4 g**

8 ounces (225 g) skinless and boneless chicken breasts

1 teaspoon five-spice powder

Low-fat cooking spray

5 ounces (150 g) prepared stir-fry vegetables (such as carrots, baby corn, cabbage, bell peppers, scallions, broccoli, bean sprouts, water chestnuts)

Grated zest and juice of 1 lemon

1 teaspoon grated peeled fresh ginger

2 tablespoons soy sauce

Salt and freshly ground black pepper

1. Cut the chicken into thin bite-size strips, and toss with the five-spice powder to coat.
2. Generously spray a wok or large nonstick frying pan with low-fat cooking spray. Heat until hot, add the chicken, and stir-fry until just cooked through, about 3 to 4 minutes. Remove with a slotted spoon and set aside.
3. Spray again, add the vegetables, and stir-fry until almost tender, about 3 to 4 minutes, depending upon selection.
4. Return the chicken to the pan with the lemon zest, lemon juice, ginger, soy sauce, and salt and pepper, mixing well. Stir-fry for 1 minute.
5. Serve hot with rice or noodles, if desired and tolerated.

Pizzafied Chicken

I know there are many early post-op and long-term bariatrics that shun carbs—some can't tolerate them; some want to watch their intake; and others avoid them because they feel they open the door to excess. I understand all of these reasons, and so I bring you an Italian-inspired dish that gives you all the taste of a cheesy pizza but none of the carby dough! This is a real deep-pan-type feast using chicken as the crust. It's wonderful both hot and cold, or am I the only one to miss and welcome back cold pizza?

○ ○ ● | SERVES **2**

PER PORTION:	CALORIES 275	PROTEIN 38.4 g	CARBOHYDRATE 18.2 g	FAT 5.9 g

Low-fat cooking spray

1 small red onion, chopped

1 garlic clove, crushed

1 green or red bell pepper, chopped

4 mushrooms, sliced (optional)

3 tomatoes, peeled and chopped

2 tablespoons tomato paste

1–2 teaspoons dried mixed herbs

Salt and freshly ground black pepper

2 skinless and boneless chicken breasts, about 4 ounces (100 g) each

1½ ounces (40 g) reduced-fat cheddar, sliced

A few fresh basil leaves

1. Preheat the oven to 425°F (220°C).
2. Spray a pan with low-fat cooking spray, heat, then add the onion, garlic, bell pepper, and mushrooms, if using. Cook for 5 to 8 minutes. Stir in the tomatoes, tomato paste, mixed herbs, and salt and pepper.
3. Meanwhile, cut each chicken breast in half horizontally to make a butterfly shape, being careful not to cut it the whole way through. The flattened chicken cooks beautifully tender compared to a whole unsliced fillet, and it's easy to cut in half later for a bariatric portion.
4. Spray a large nonstick sauté pan with low-fat cooking spray, heat, add the chicken, and cook on both sides over high heat, until golden. Transfer to a baking sheet and bake for 15 to 20 minutes, until just tender.
5. Top the chicken with the prepared tomato mixture, arrange the cheese on top, and sprinkle with a few basil leaves. Return to the oven for 5 minutes so that the cheese just melts. Serve hot with vegetables or salad, or cold with a salad, as desired.

Ultimate Bariatric Shepherd's Pie

WLS
PORTION:
½

This is the ultimate shepherd's pie. Why? Because it has a superb, creamy, low-carb topping that rivals mashed potatoes any day. It's arguably richer and tastier and no one notices the difference. It's suitable for the Soft Food (Yellow) stage of eating and thereafter, and the portion size can be increased as time goes on. I use special bariatric Portion, Cook, and Serve measuring cups to make mine, so that I can make just the right amount. You can substitute with your own small bakeware, and small ramekins will also suffice.

○ ◐ ●		SERVES 6		✱

PER PORTION:	CALORIES 300	PROTEIN 33.1 g	CARBOHYDRATE 22.1 g	FAT 7.9 g

1 medium cauliflower, cut into large pieces
(about 4 to 6 cups)

2 teaspoons olive oil

Two 11-ounce (300 g) cans cooked white beans
(cannellini, for example), drained
and rinsed

Salt and freshly ground black pepper

1½ pounds (700 g) lean ground beef, lamb, or
turkey

1 large onion, finely chopped

2 garlic cloves, crushed

14-ounce (400 g) can diced tomatoes or 1-pound
(500 g) carton passata (crushed tomatoes)

2-3 tablespoons Worcestershire sauce

¼ cup (65 g) tomato paste

1 beef bouillon cube, crumbled

Sliced tomatoes, to top (optional)

1. **To make the cauliflower mash,** place the cauliflower in a pan and add sufficient water to just cover. Bring to a boil, reduce the heat, and simmer until fork-tender, about 10 minutes. Drain well, then transfer to a blender with the oil, beans, and salt and pepper. Blend until smooth and set aside.

2. Preheat the oven to 300°F (150°C).

3. Cook the beef or lamb in a nonstick, lidded, ovenproof pan until browned. Add the onion and garlic and cook for 5 to 10 minutes, until softened.

4. Add the tomatoes or passata, Worcestershire sauce, tomato paste, bouillon cube, and salt and pepper, mixing well. Cook for 5 minutes.

5. Cover and cook in the oven for 1 hour, then increase the oven temperature to 400°F (200°C).

6. Transfer the meat mixture to a suitable ovenproof dish or divide into small individual baking dishes and top with the prepared cauliflower and bean mash. Top with sliced tomatoes, if desired.

7. Bake for 20 to 30 minutes, until golden brown. Serve hot.

Super Speedy Chili in a Shell

WLS PORTION: ½

When the weather turns cooler, we always turn to chili for a fail-safe warming main meal. It's easy to make well ahead, is time- and temperature-tolerant, feeds a crowd, and is bariatric-friendly. Lately, I have been serving ours in crisp taco shells instead of with rice (but still with the usual toppings). That way those who can't tolerate rice don't have to leave theirs and those who want to avoid carbs can eat the filling and ignore the "container."

○ ● ●		SERVES **4**		✳
PER PORTION (without taco shells and toppings):	CALORIES **285**	PROTEIN **33 g**	CARBOHYDRATE **24.7 g**	FAT **5.9 g**

1 pound (500 g) extra-lean ground beef

1 large onion, chopped

One 14-ounce (400 g) can diced tomatoes

1 red or green chile, seeded and chopped (optional)

1 beef bouillon cube

1 tablespoon Worcestershire sauce

Salt and freshly ground black pepper

One 14-ounce (400 g) can chili beans (red kidney beans in a chili sauce)

8 tortillas, to make crisp taco shells (optional)

1. Cook the beef in a large nonstick frying pan, breaking it up with a spoon, until browned, about 7 minutes.
2. Add the onion and cook for 3 to 5 more minutes.
3. Add the tomatoes, chile, if using, bouillon cube, Worcestershire sauce, and salt and pepper, mixing well. Cover and cook for 10 minutes.
4. Add the chili beans, mixing well, cover and cook for 10 minutes, until tender.
5. Serve with rice, if desired, or prepare the crisp taco shells as below. Top with the usual accompaniments, like guacamole and grated cheese, if desired.

TO MAKE CRISP TACO SHELLS: Heat tortillas until warm—this prevents them from cracking and breaking. Here are 3 ways.

A. **In the oven:** Wrap stacks of 8 tortillas in foil and place in a 375°F (190°C) oven for 10 to 15 minutes.

B. **On the stove top:** Turn the burner on high. Using tongs, slide one tortilla at a time over the burner for a few seconds, alternating sides, until it softens and begins to char. Cover tortillas to keep warm.

C. **In the microwave:** Wrap a stack of 8 tortillas in a barely damp, clean kitchen towel (or paper towel); microwave for 30 to 45 seconds.

TO COOK: Preheat the oven to 375°F (190°C). Heat the tortillas until warm (see above). Coat each side with low-fat cooking spray. Turn a muffin pan upside down. Nestle a tortilla in the space between 4 cups to form a bowl. Repeat with 3 more tortillas, making 4 bowls in total. Bake until firm and beginning to brown, about 15 minutes. Transfer to a wire rack to cool. Repeat with the remaining 4 tortillas.

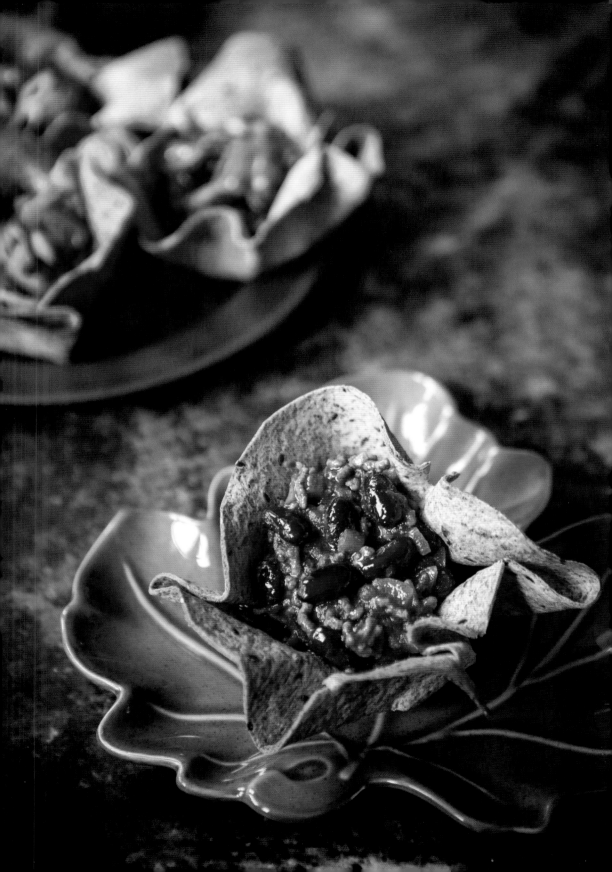

Moroccan Beef with Couscous and Zucchini

Extra-lean ground beef makes a great meal after WLS, and in this recipe it is cooked with onion, garlic, red bell peppers, and a Moroccan spice called *ras el hanout*. It's a spice mixture used throughout North Africa and literally translates to "top of the shop"—a spice mix with the best of all in its make-up. Mine had chiles, rose petals, and ginger, among other fragrant spices. It makes for a fabulously fragrant beef mixture to serve with couscous and charred zucchini.

○ ○ ● | SERVES **4**

PER PORTION:	CALORIES **450**	PROTEIN **39.3 g**	CARBOHYDRATE **56.8 g**	FAT **7.5 g**

1 pound (500 g) extra-lean ground beef

2 red onions, chopped

2 red bell peppers, cored, seeded, and thinly sliced

2 tablespoons ras el hanout

2 garlic cloves, crushed

Salt and freshly ground black pepper

Two 14-ounce (400 g) cans diced tomatoes

2 beef bouillon cubes

1 generous cup (200 g) couscous

2 zucchini, sliced

Large bunch cilantro, chopped

A few toasted sliced almonds, to serve

1. Cook the beef in a large nonstick frying pan over high heat, breaking it up with a spoon, until browned, about 7 minutes.
2. Add the onion, bell peppers, and ras el hanout, mixing well. Cook for 5 minutes. Add the garlic and salt and pepper and cook for 1 minute.
3. Add the tomatoes, bouillon cubes, and ⅔ cup (150 ml) water. Bring to a boil, then reduce the heat to medium-low and cook for about 20 minutes.
4. About 10 minutes before the end of cooking, place the couscous in a bowl and cover with 2 cups (400 ml) boiling water (or follow the package instructions). Cover and let stand for 10 minutes.
5. Meanwhile, heat a large cast-iron skillet over medium heat without any oil, and cook the zucchini slices, 5 minutes on each side, until nicely charred in appearance—you may have to do this in 2 batches. Keep warm.
6. To serve, stir the cilantro into the beef mixture. Fluff the couscous with a fork to separate the grains and divide among serving plates. Top with the beef mixture and charred zucchini, then sprinkle with a few almonds to serve.

Sweet Potato Cottage Pie

Who doesn't love a cottage pie? Wonderfully comforting and warming on a chilly day . . . it has the virtue of being easily prepared well ahead (and freezes beautifully) for relaxed eating. Since surgery, I've been making mine with a sweet potato topping (for lower GI carbs). I love the color contrast between the dark meaty base and the golden topping. It makes a great one-dish family meal but can be made in small individual ramekins, if preferred. Sometimes I like to serve it with a crisp vegetable and other times I serve with a slice or two of avocado and a sprinkling of fresh basil on top.

○ ◐ ●		SERVES **4**		✱
PER PORTION (without optional toppings):	CALORIES **360**	PROTEIN **33.1 g**	CARBOHYDRATE **40.7 g**	FAT **7.6 g**

Low-fat cooking spray

1 onion, finely chopped

1 carrot, finely chopped

2 stalks celery, finely chopped

1 pound (500 g) extra-lean ground beef

2 tablespoons Worcestershire sauce

2 tablespoons tomato paste

14-ounce (400 g) can diced tomatoes

1 teaspoon dried mixed herbs

²/₃ cup (100 g) frozen peas

Salt and freshly ground black pepper

2 large sweet potatoes (about 1¼ pounds/600 g), peeled and chopped

2 to 3 tablespoons low-fat milk

1 ounce (30 g) reduced-fat feta cheese, crumbled

Sliced avocado and torn basil leaves, to top (optional)

1. Preheat the oven to 350°F (180°C).
2. Generously spray a pan with low-fat cooking spray. Heat, add the onion, carrot, and celery, and cook, stirring, for 3 to 4 minutes, until softened. Add the beef and cook, stirring to break up the meat, for 5 to 8 minutes, or until browned.
3. Add the Worcestershire sauce, tomato paste, tomatoes, and herbs. Bring to a boil, reduce the heat to low, and simmer for 20 to 25 minutes, or until reduced and thickened. Stir in the peas and salt and pepper.
4. Meanwhile, cook the sweet potato in boiling salted water until just tender, about 8 to 10 minutes. Drain, return to the pan, add the milk, and mash until smooth.
5. Spoon the beef mixture into one large baking dish or individual ramekins. Top with the sweet potato mixture and sprinkle with the feta. Bake for 30 to 35 minutes, or until golden.
6. Serve topped with slices of avocado and torn basil leaves, if desired, or with an additional seasonal vegetable.

Beef and Apple Meatballs

I frequently make my own meatballs and flavor them with herbs, spices, and other seasonings according to the weather, what's in season, and what tickles the taste buds on a particular day. Sometimes we have lamb meatballs flavored with mint and harissa paste, other times pork with sage and chopped yellow bell pepper, but most often it's beef ones. Beef is also the choice here, with coarsely grated apple and sage and cooked in a simple sauce made from passata. Serve with some freshly cooked pasta if you can tolerate it, or zucchini "pasta" ribbons if you can't.

○ ○ ●	SERVES **4**	✳

PER PORTION:	CALORIES **301**	PROTEIN **29.2 g**	CARBOHYDRATE **30.3 g**	FAT **7.1 g**

1 pound (450 g, about 3) apples (such as Gala or Granny Smith), peeled, cored, and quartered

1 pound (450 g) extra-lean ground beef

1½ cups (75 g) soft fresh bread crumbs

1 tablespoon chopped fresh sage

1 egg yolk, beaten

Salt and freshly ground black pepper

Low-fat cooking spray

1 pound (700 g) passata (crushed tomatoes) with onion and garlic

1. Coarsely grate the apples and place half in a large bowl. Add the beef, bread crumbs, sage, egg yolk, and salt and pepper. Use clean hands to mix the ingredients together, then divide and shape into about 32 small meatballs.

2. Generously spray a large nonstick frying or sauté pan with low-fat cooking spray. Heat, add the meatballs, and fry over a high heat for about 6 to 8 minutes, stirring and turning occasionally, until golden brown on all sides.

3. Add the remaining grated apple and stir well. Add the passata and salt and pepper. Cover and simmer for 5 to 7 minutes, or until the sauce has thickened slightly and the meatballs are cooked through.

4. Serve hot with freshly cooked pasta, if desired.

Slow-Cooked Lamb and Bean Stew

WLS
PORTION:
½

This is a simple but hearty one-pot supper that's perfect for making ahead. It doesn't need any additional accompaniments but those who are not following a strict WLS regimen (and can tolerate it) may like a little rustic bread to mop up the juices.

○ ● ● | SERVES **4**

| PER PORTION: | CALORIES **365** | PROTEIN **29.9 g** | CARBOHYDRATE **43.1 g** | FAT **7.6 g** |

Low-fat cooking spray

12 ounces (350 g) diced lean lamb

2 slices lean bacon, coarsely chopped

2 onions, chopped

1 celery stalk, chopped

1 carrot, chopped

2 garlic cloves, chopped

1 teaspoon fennel seeds

2 russet potatoes (about 16 ounces/500 g), peeled and chopped

14-ounce (400 g) can borlotti beans, drained and rinsed

2 tablespoons double-concentrated tomato paste

Scant 2 cups (500 ml) beef stock

Salt and freshly ground black pepper

8 ounces (250 g) spinach leaves

1. Generously spray a large, deep pan with low-fat cooking spray. Heat, add the lamb, bacon, onions, celery, and carrot and cook for 5 to 10 minutes, until lightly browned.

2. Add the garlic and fennel seeds and cook for 1 minute.

3. Stir in the potatoes, beans, tomato paste, stock, and season with salt and pepper. Cover and simmer gently for about 50 minutes, or until the lamb is tender.

4. Stir in the spinach, cook for 1 to 2 minutes, until wilted, then ladle into bowls to serve.

NOTE: If you are at the early onset of the Soft Food (Yellow) stage, feel free to purée or fork-mash the entire recipe to a suitable texture and consistency.

Speedy Summer Lamb Tagine

Summer food doesn't always have to be about barbecues, grills, and salads—there are a whole host of dishes that can be quickly cooked for a flavorful meal. Here's one—lamb quickly cooked with beans, tomatoes, and a few soft dried apricots—delicious served with couscous.

SERVES 4			
PER PORTION:	CALORIES **543**	PROTEIN **40.3 g**	CARBOHYDRATE **79.8 g**	FAT **7.7 g**

Low-fat cooking spray

1 red onion, sliced

1 pound (450 g) diced lean leg of lamb

Salt and freshly ground black pepper

1 green chile, seeded and thinly sliced (optional)

11 ounces (300 g) tomatoes, roughly chopped

14-ounce (400 g) can cannellini beans, drained and
  rinsed

8 soft dried apricots, quartered

2½ cups (600 ml) hot beef stock

1¾ cups (300 g) couscous

Grated zest and juice of 1 lemon

Chopped fresh cilantro leaves, to garnish

1. Generously spray a large frying or sauté pan with low-fat cooking spray. Heat, add the onion and lamb, season with salt and pepper, and stir-fry for 5 minutes.
2. Add the chile, if using, and tomatoes and cook for 5 minutes, or until the tomatoes are softened.
3. Stir in the cannellini beans, apricots, and a quarter of the stock. Simmer for 10 minutes.
4. Meanwhile, place the couscous in a large heatproof bowl with the lemon zest and juice and cover with the remaining hot stock. Cover and set aside for 5 minutes, until all the liquid has been absorbed.
5. Break up the couscous with a fork and divide between serving bowls. Top with the lamb tagine and scatter with the cilantro to serve.

NOTE: If you are at the early onset of the Soft Food (Yellow) stage, feel free to purée or fork-mash the entire recipe to a suitable texture and consistency.

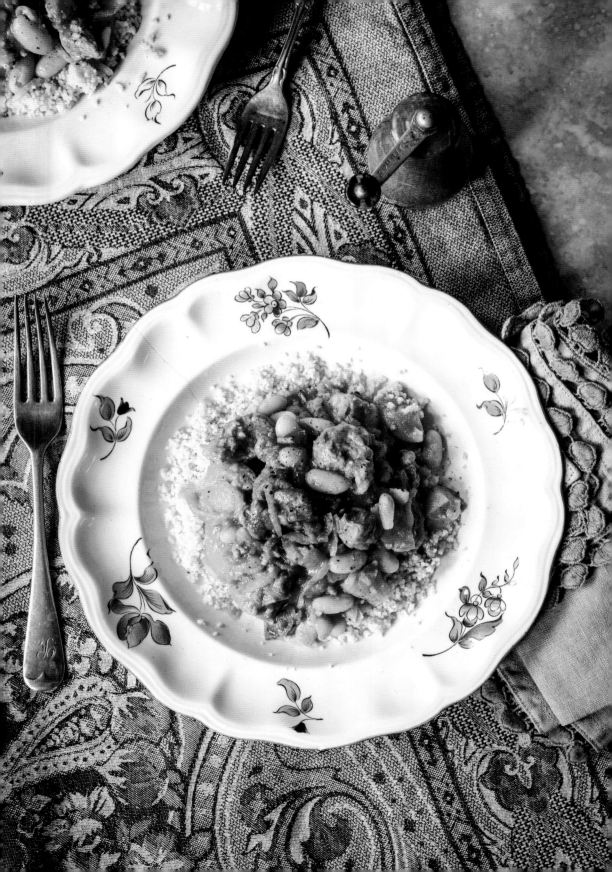

Slow-Cooked Spiced Pork

Pork, dried fruit, and spices make a heavenly stew to enjoy in autumn and winter. This one has a wonderful fruity and spicy flavor from the addition of dates, apricots, and mellow spices, like cinnamon, mace, and just a hint of mild curry powder. You could serve this with potatoes, rice, or couscous—whatever you like and can tolerate. A side dish of shredded cabbage would also be welcome. You can prepare this in the conventional oven or in a slow cooker. If you like a stew with a thicker consistency, just add a little cornstarch dissolved in cold water toward the end of the cooking time.

		SERVES 6		
PER PORTION:	CALORIES **235**	PROTEIN **28.9 g**	CARBOHYDRATE **25.5 g**	FAT **2.1 g**

Low-fat cooking spray

1¾ pounds (800 g) stewing pork or pork leg, diced

1 large onion, sliced

3 stalks celery, sliced

2 garlic cloves, crushed

1 teaspoon ground cinnamon

1 teaspoon ground mace

1 teaspoon mild curry powder

2 tablespoons chopped fresh thyme

⅔ cup (100 g) chopped soft dried dates

⅔ cup (100 g) chopped soft dried apricots

Grated zest and juice of 1 orange

2 cups (450 ml) vegetable stock

Salt and freshly ground black pepper

2 tablespoons chopped fresh parsley

1. Preheat the oven to 325°F (170°C).
2. Spray a large nonstick sauté pan with low-fat cooking spray. Heat, add the pork, and cook on all sides, until browned. Transfer with a slotted spoon to a baking dish.
3. Add the onion, celery, garlic, cinnamon, mace, and curry powder to the pan juices and cook for 3 to 4 minutes, stirring frequently.
4. Add the thyme, dates, apricots, orange zest and juice, and stock, mixing well. Season well with salt and pepper and bring to a boil. Pour over the pork in the baking dish, cover, and bake for 1½ to 2 hours, until the pork is tender.
5. Sprinkle the parsley over the top to serve.

NOTE: If you are at the early onset of the Soft Food (Yellow) stage, feel free to purée or fork-mash the entire recipe to a suitable texture and consistency.

TO COOK IN A SLOW COOKER: Prepare as above but reduce the stock to 1¼ cups (300 ml). Place the browned pork and vegetable/fruit mixture in a slow cooker and cook on high for 1 hour. Reduce the cooker setting to low and cook for an additional 3 to 4 hours, until the pork is very tender. Finish for serving as above.

Cupboard Chorizo and Bean Hotpot

This is one of those very handy cupboard recipes that makes the best of some canned food and takes just half an hour to prepare, cook, and serve. It's the sort of dish to make when you don't want to go out shopping, find yourself at the month's end and the purse strings are tight, or simply looking for something nutritious to cook in a hurry. It's perfect comfort food that is cheap and cheerful and yet has a warming spicy kick. You will need a cured chorizo sausage, but it's worth keeping one in the refrigerator just for this recipe. Serve with a little crusty bread if you can tolerate it.

SERVES **4**

PER PORTION:	CALORIES **270**	PROTEIN **16.6 g**	CARBOHYDRATE **31.6 g**	FAT **8.8 g**

4 ounces (125 g) cured chorizo sausage, skinned and chopped

3 red onions, chopped

3 garlic cloves, crushed

1 teaspoon smoked paprika

14-ounce (400 g) can diced tomatoes

Two 14-ounce (400 g) cans lima beans, drained and rinsed

Salt and freshly ground black pepper

1. Cook the chorizo, onions, and garlic in a large frying pan until the oil begins to run. Continue to sauté over a gentle heat, stirring occasionally, until the onions are soft.
2. Add the smoked paprika, tomatoes, and lima beans, mixing well. Stir and simmer over low heat for about 10 minutes.
3. Season to taste with salt and pepper, then spoon into dishes to serve, with bread to mop up the spicy juices, if desired.

NOTE: If you are at the early onset of the Soft Food (Yellow) stage, feel free to purée or fork-mash the entire recipe to a suitable texture and consistency.

Campfire-Style Sausage and Beans

WLS PORTION: ½

This is a regular mid-week family favorite, and we never tire of it because I use different sausages and beans. All I insist upon are good-quality, low-fat, high-protein sausages (ideally with at least 85 percent meat). As for the beans, baked beans are great, but this dish is lifted into the luxury class if you use barbecue baked beans, curried beans, or some of the special canned recipe ones like Tuscan- or fajita-style. Hearty appetites might enjoy a spoonful of mashed potatoes or couscous to mop up the juices.

○ ○ ● | SERVES **4**

PER PORTION:	CALORIES **220**	PROTEIN **22 g**	CARBOHYDRATE **21.5 g**	FAT **3.4 g**

Low-fat cooking spray

6 to 8 low-fat, high–meat content sausages
(weighing about 1 pound/450 g)

2 red onions, finely chopped

2 stalks celery, finely chopped

14-ounce (400 g) can diced tomatoes

2/3 cup (150 ml) vegetable stock

2 bay leaves

15-ounce (415 g) can baked beans, or flavored
beans in sauce

Salt and freshly ground black pepper

Chopped parsley, to garnish

1. Generously spray a large nonstick sauté pan with low-fat cooking spray. Heat, then add the sausages, and cook over medium heat, until browned on all sides. Remove from the pan and set aside.

2. Add the red onion and celery to the pan and cook over low heat, until softened, about 5 minutes.

3. Add the tomatoes, stock, and bay leaves. Cook over low heat for 10 minutes, stirring occasionally.

4. Return the sausages to the pan with the beans and salt and pepper, mixing well. Cook over low heat for about 10 to 15 minutes, until the sausages are fully cooked and fork tender and the sauce has thickened slightly. Discard the bay leaves.

5. Serve hot, garnished with chopped parsley, and with mashed potatoes or couscous, if desired.

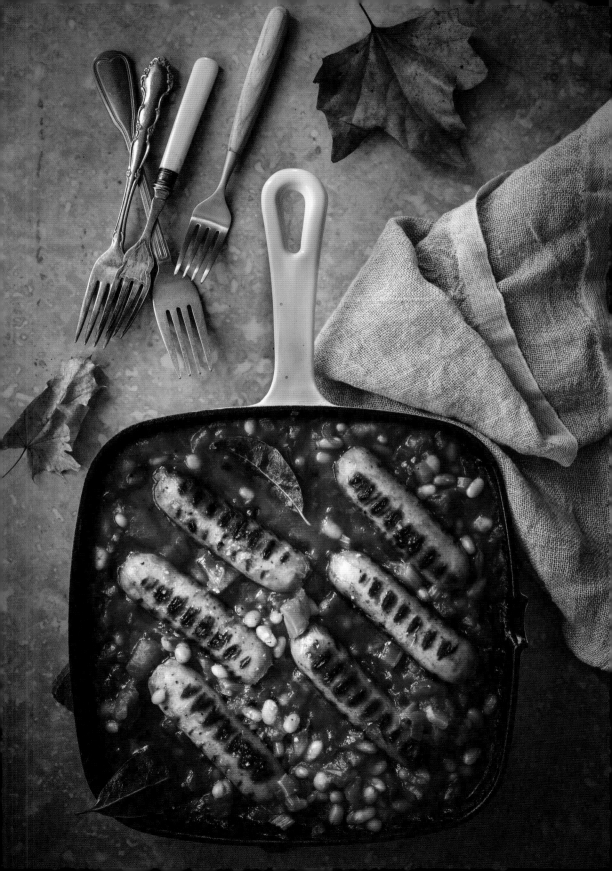

Ricotta Bake

In weight loss surgery forums and groups, this is a recipe that is passed around frequently—and there are a few variations of it. Why is it so popular? Because it's a dish that has a soft texture and consistency, which allows it to be eaten and enjoyed soon after surgery; it's flavorful when you are tired of bland food; it has a good high-protein profile, with over 15 g per WLS portion; and leftovers reheat well (in the microwave). Non-WLS diners enjoy it with a salad, too—so it's a win-win!

○ ◐ ●	SERVES 2	Ⓥ

PER PORTION:	CALORIES 358	PROTEIN 31 g	CARBOHYDRATE 8.7 g	FAT 22.6 g

8 ounces (225 g) ricotta

½ cup (50 g) grated Parmesan cheese

1 large egg, beaten

1 teaspoon dried Italian herb seasoning

Salt and freshly ground black pepper

½ cup (125 g) pasta sauce

½ cup (50 g) grated reduced-fat mozzarella cheese

1. Preheat the oven to 425°F (220°C).
2. Mix the ricotta, Parmesan, egg, Italian seasoning, and salt and pepper. Pour into a baking dish.
3. Spoon the pasta sauce on top and sprinkle with the mozzarella cheese. Bake for 20 to 25 minutes.
4. Allow to cool slightly before serving.

Mixed Bean Chili

WLS PORTION: ½

This mixed bean chili is ideal for vegetarians—but, that said, a spoonful is also wonderful alongside a piece of grilled chicken or steak; and you could add chopped cooked meat to it, if you wish. It's even delicious cold, like a bean salad, and I have used it as a filling for an omelet. The instructions below refer to cooking it on the stove top, but you can prepare in a slow cooker, too. Cook on high for 2 hours, and then low for 2 to 3 hours—and if you want a thicker mixture, leave it only partially covered for the last hour of cooking.

○ ◐ ●	SERVES 4	Ⓥ	✳
PER PORTION:	CALORIES **262**	PROTEIN **14.2 g**	CARBOHYDRATE **42.9 g**	FAT **3.1 g**

Low-fat cooking spray

1 onion, finely chopped

2 garlic cloves, crushed

1 carrot, peeled and chopped (optional)

1 yellow, red, or orange bell pepper, cored, seeded, and chopped

14-ounce (400 g) can diced tomatoes

1 vegetable bouillon cube

1 teaspoon ground cumin

1 teaspoon ground cinnamon

1 teaspoon mild chili powder

14-ounce (400 g) can red kidney beans in chili sauce

14-ounce (400 g) can beans (black-eyed peas, black beans, navy beans, lima beans, or a mixture), drained and rinsed

4 ounces (100 g) cooked corn

Sprig of fresh rosemary and thyme, chopped

Salt and freshly ground black pepper

Cilantro, to garnish (optional)

1. Generously spray a large, deep pan with low-fat cooking spray. Heat, add the onion, garlic, carrot, if using, and bell pepper. Cook for 2 to 3 minutes, stirring frequently.

2. Add the tomatoes, bouillon cube, cumin, cinnamon, and chili powder, and bring to a boil. Reduce the heat, cover, and simmer for 10 minutes, until the vegetables are tender.

3. Add all the beans, the corn, herbs, and season with salt and pepper, mixing well. Cook for about 10 minutes, until the beans are hot and the mixture has reduced and thickened slightly.

4. Serve hot with rice, if tolerated, or cold as an accompaniment, sprinkled with cilantro, if desired.

NOTE: If you are at the early onset of the Soft Food (Yellow) stage, feel free to purée or fork-mash the entire recipe to a suitable texture and consistency.

Quick and Simple Vegetable Stir-Fry

My family calls this "health on a plate." I make it a few times a month, when time is limited and I need to make a meal from whatever vegetables lurk in my refrigerator. One of our favorites uses mushrooms, Napa cabbage, baby corn, and red bell peppers, but it will work just as well with vegetables like thinly sliced carrots, leeks, broccoli florets, green beans, and scallions—in other words, whatever is at hand. The short cooking time means it's on the table in minutes but it also allows the vegetables to retain all their goodness. A WLS patient will find this meal ideal quantity-wise for a main dish, but add noodles or rice for those who haven't had surgery, to satisfy their larger appetites.

○ ○ ● | SERVES **4** | **V**

PER PORTION:	CALORIES **125**	PROTEIN **8.9 g**	CARBOHYDRATE **13.9 g**	FAT **4 g**

2 teaspoons sesame oil, or low-fat cooking spray

2 garlic cloves, crushed

1 chile, finely chopped

1 onion, sliced

1 pound (500 g) mushrooms, sliced or halved

1 pound (500 g) Napa cabbage, coarsely chopped or shredded

11 ounces (300 g) canned baby corn, halved lengthwise

2 red bell peppers, cored, seeded, and sliced

¼ cup soy sauce

Small handful chopped cilantro (optional)

1. Place the oil in a large wok or pan, or generously spray the pan with low-fat cooking spray, then heat to hot.
2. Add the garlic and chile and cook for 30 seconds.
3. Add the onion, mushrooms, Napa cabbage, baby corn, and bell peppers, and stir-fry for about 4 minutes, or until tender-crisp.
4. Add the soy sauce, mixing and tossing well.
5. Spoon into serving bowls and sprinkle with the cilantro, if using, to serve.

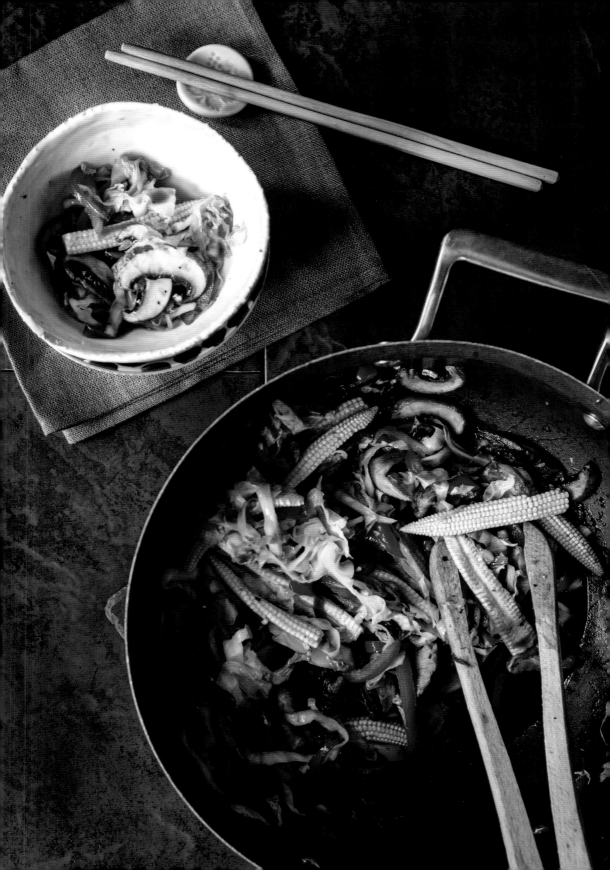

Eggplant Parmesan

WLS PORTION:
½–1

Every now and again, I try a recipe revamp (to make it bariatric-friendly) and it blows me away when it's better. This is one of them! The classic northern Italian eggplant Parmesan, usually made with vegetables, tomato sauce, and cheese, is also highly calorific—but cooked this new way, it isn't. I have made it with tofu alone, but also with tofu and ground beef, or with beef alone. All variations work superbly, so decide for yourself whether you want the vegetarian or the carnivore option, or the half-and-half one. You can also use Quorn. If using the meat, simply brown in a pan until no longer pink. You can speed up this recipe by using frozen eggplant and zucchini, so there will be no need to precook at all. You'll need about 1½ pounds (750 g).

○ ● ●	SERVES **4** (generously)	✳
PER PORTION (with tofu/ tofu and beef/beef alone):		

	CALORIES	PROTEIN	CARBOHYDRATE	FAT
	327/353/383	28.3 g/30.6 g/33.2 g	16.1 g/15.3 g/14.5 g	17.1 g/19 g/21.1 g

1 eggplant (about 1 pound / 450 g)

Low-fat cooking spray

Salt and freshly ground black pepper

1 pound (450 g) firm tofu, or tofu and cooked ground beef, or cooked ground beef

1 cup (100 g) shredded low-fat mozzarella cheese

1 cup (250 g) reduced-fat ricotta cheese

2 cups (450 g) low-sugar tomato sauce

Large handful of fresh basil leaves

1 large zucchini, sliced into thin rounds

3 tablespoons grated Parmesan cheese

Fresh basil sprigs, to garnish (optional)

1. Preheat the oven to 425°F (220°C).
2. Slice the eggplant into ¼-inch (6 mm) discs and place in a single layer on a nonstick baking sheet (you may need 2 sheets) and spray liberally with low-fat cooking spray. Season with salt and pepper and bake, until lightly browned and tender, about 15 minutes. Remove and set aside.
3. Meanwhile, if using the tofu, squeeze firmly to remove as much liquid as possible, then crumble into a bowl. If using beef, add to the tofu, or place the whole quantity into a bowl if using beef alone. Add the mozzarella and ricotta cheeses and season with salt and pepper, mixing well.
4. Cover the bottom of a 9 x 12 inch (23 x 30 cm) baking dish with about ¾ cup (175 g) of the tomato sauce. Top with half of the basil leaves torn into rough pieces, then half of the baked eggplant, half of the zucchini rounds and, finally, half of the tofu or beef mixture.
5. Repeat with an additional ¾ cup (175 ml) of the tomato sauce, the remaining basil, baked eggplant, zucchini, and tofu or beef mixture. Finally, spoon over the remaining tomato sauce and sprinkle with the Parmesan cheese. At this stage, the dish can be covered and chilled until required for cooking.
6. Bake the prepared dish, until the eggplant is tender and the dish is golden and crusty on top, about 30 to 40 minutes.
7. Let stand for 5 minutes after removing from the oven before slicing to serve, garnished with basil, if desired.

NOTE: If you are at the early onset of the Soft Food (Yellow) stage, feel free to purée or fork-mash the entire recipe to a suitable texture and consistency.

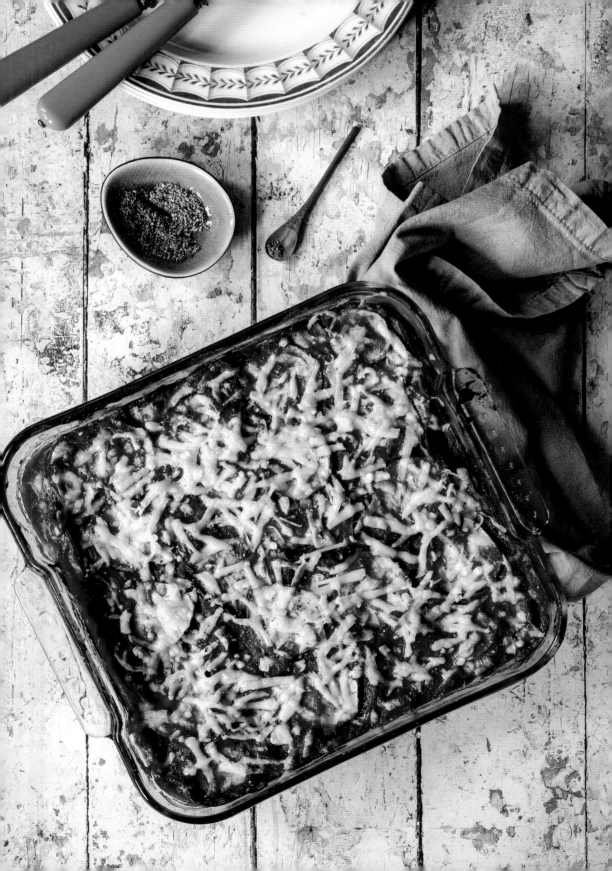

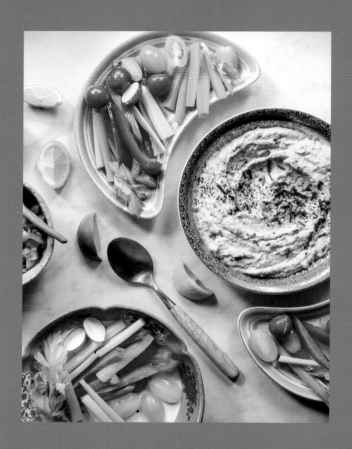

Vegetables, Dips, and Side Dishes

———

Holiday Crunch Red Cabbage and Apple Slaw

I call this "Holiday" because that's when I tend to serve this slaw—at Christmas, Thanksgiving, Easter, or a national holiday celebration. It goes so well with deli fare and other buffet-style table offerings. It beats any ready-made coleslaw you might find. It's light, colorful, and has sufficient crunch to make the dreariest of leftovers sing with flavor. For those who like them, a few dried cranberries can be added to the mix for a measured sweet extra and festive touch.

○ ○ ●	SERVES **4**	**V**

PER PORTION:	CALORIES **108**	PROTEIN **3.7 g**	CARBOHYDRATE **11.2 g**	FAT **5.2 g**

8 ounces (225 g) red cabbage, finely shredded

2 carrots, peeled and coarsely grated

1 red apple, cored, sliced, and tossed in a little lemon juice

¼ cup (25 g) pecans or walnuts

7-ounce (200 g) bag salad greens

¼ cup (65 g) low-fat plain yogurt

Grated zest and juice of 1 lemon

Salt and freshly ground black pepper

1. Mix the red cabbage with the carrots, apple, pecans or walnuts, and salad greens in a serving bowl, and toss to mix.
2. Mix the yogurt with the lemon zest, lemon juice, and salt and pepper. Drizzle over the slaw to serve.

Strawberry Jar Salad

I love to make mason jar salads to take along on picnics because they travel well, make a great side dish (or even main dish) to mix and match with other portable fare, and can be easily personalized according to likes and dislikes. This one seems to be enjoyed by just about everyone and is a firm favorite. The fruitiness of the strawberries with the sharpness of the mint and the saltiness of the feta seems to hit all the right notes. You will need a pint-size (500 g) mason jar or equivalent for the normal-size portion of this recipe—about half this size for a WLS portion.

○ ○ ●	SERVES 1	Ⓥ
PER PORTION:	CALORIES **415**	PROTEIN **15.3 g**	CARBOHYDRATE **36.2 g**	FAT **22.5 g**

1 tablespoon balsamic vinegar

1 tablespoon olive oil

Salt and freshly ground black pepper

1 cup (100 g) canned chickpeas, rinsed and drained

A handful of arugula

1½ cups (250 g) strawberries, hulled and quartered

1 ounce (25 g) feta cheese, cubed

1 tablespoon chopped fresh mint

Juice of ½ lemon

1. Pour the balsamic vinegar and oil into the jar. Season with salt and pepper and shake to mix.

2. Layer the chickpeas, arugula, strawberries, feta, and mint in the jar. It is important not to have the salad leaves next to the dressing as the vinegar will cause them to go limp. Seal the jar.

3. When ready to eat, add the lemon juice, shake the jar to coat the salad, and enjoy straight from the jar, or tip onto a plate to serve. Store upright and chill until serving.

Rule the Roast Vegetables

I simply adore roast vegetables and think I could eat them for almost any meal. There is a version for any season. I use a combination of root vegetables in the winter months; early baby ones mixed with late winter tubers in the springtime; kitchen garden favorites in all their glory in the summer when I tire of salads; and colorful squashes, bell peppers, and tomatoes in the autumn. All mixed and matched with herbs, spices, and flavorings to suit. Below is my basic late summer to autumn one, with squash or pumpkin, bell peppers, zucchini, eggplant, onions, garlic, and herbs. It's very tasty and can be made into a main meal if you top it with slices of halloumi cheese and sprinkle with pine nuts for the last twenty minutes of cooking.

	SERVES 4		Ⓥ
PER PORTION:	CALORIES 106	PROTEIN 4 g	CARBOHYDRATE 21.3 g	FAT 1.1 g

1 medium butternut squash

2 red bell peppers

2 red onions

1 zucchini, thickly sliced

1 small eggplant, cubed

Low-fat cooking spray

2 garlic cloves, crushed

2 tablespoons fresh mixed chopped herbs of your choice (basil, rosemary, and thyme)

Salt and freshly ground black pepper

1 tablespoon balsamic vinegar

1. Preheat the oven to 400°F (200°C).
2. Peel the squash, cut it in half lengthwise, and remove any seeds. Cut the flesh into chunks and place in a large nonstick roasting pan.
3. Cut the bell peppers in half, remove the seeds and stems, and cut into chunky pieces. Add to the pan.
4. Peel and halve the onions, cut into small wedges, and add to the pan with the zucchini and eggplant.
5. Spray generously with low-fat cooking spray, add the garlic and herbs, and season with salt and pepper. Toss well to coat. Roast for 45 to 50 minutes, or until slightly charred around the edges and tender.
6. Add the balsamic vinegar and toss to mix. Serve hot, or let cool and serve cold.

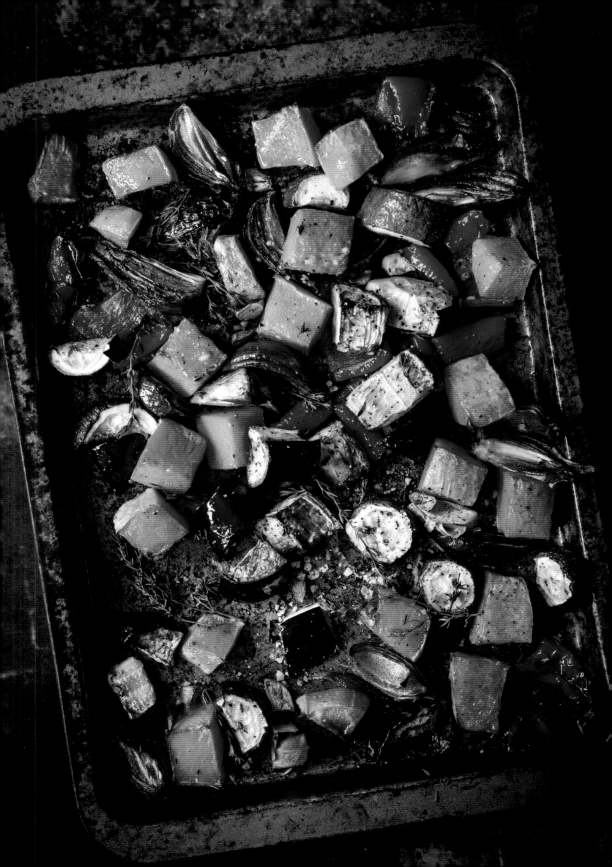

Griddled Zucchini with Mint

These zucchini are bursting with herby spring flavors and taste wonderful with roasted salmon and other baked fish. This recipe also works well with thinly sliced fennel.

		SERVES 4		Ⓥ
PER PORTION:	CALORIES 70	PROTEIN 3.4 g	CARBOHYDRATE 3.5 g	FAT 4.8 g

1 pound (500 g) zucchini

1 small garlic clove, crushed

1 tablespoon extra virgin olive oil

Grated zest and juice of 1 lemon

1 mild green chile, seeded and finely chopped

1 tablespoon grated Parmesan cheese

3 tablespoons chopped fresh mint

Salt and freshly ground black pepper

1. Cut the zucchini into ¼-inch (6 mm) slices lengthwise and place in a large bowl with the garlic and oil. Toss gently to coat.
2. Cook the zucchini slices in a hot grill pan (or on a barbecue), turning frequently, until tender and lightly charred.
3. Remove to a serving plate and scatter with the lemon zest, lemon juice, and chile. Cover and let cool and marinate until ready to serve, or serve immediately, while still hot.
4. Just before serving, scatter with the Parmesan, mint, and season with salt and pepper. Toss gently to mix and serve.

Asparagus with Lime and Sour Cream Glaze

Here's an asparagus dish that makes a great starter, light lunch, or accompaniment at a barbecue. The spice seasoning is mild but you can add a little more or less to suit your taste.

○ ○ ●	SERVES **2**	**V**

PER PORTION:	CALORIES **100**	PROTEIN **8.7 g**	CARBOHYDRATE **4.8 g**	FAT **5.2 g**

12-ounce (320 g) bunch asparagus, trimmed
Low-fat cooking spray
1 tablespoon sour cream
Juice of ½ lime
Scant ¼ cup (20 g) finely grated Parmesan cheese
½ teaspoon chili powder
½ teaspoon ground cumin

1. Generously spray the asparagus with low-fat cooking spray and cook on a hot grill pan for 5 minutes, turning regularly.
2. Meanwhile, combine the sour cream with the lime juice and, in a separate bowl, mix the Parmesan with the chili powder and cumin.
3. Once the asparagus is cooked, brush each spear with the sour cream mixture, then sprinkle with the Parmesan mixture to serve.

Peas with Brussels Sprouts in an Orange Nut Glaze

Love them or loathe them, Brussels sprouts have divided popularity. This twist on serving them with peas and a lovely orangey and nutty glaze might just sway any doubters!

	SERVES **6**		**V**
PER PORTION:	CALORIES **147**	PROTEIN **6.6 g**	CARBOHYDRATE **10.3 g**	FAT **8.8 g**

7 ounces (200 g) small Brussels sprouts, trimmed

14 ounces (400 g) frozen peas

¼ cup (55 g) light butter, or low-fat spread

½ cup (50 g) chopped hazelnuts

Grated zest and juice of 1 orange

Salt and freshly ground black pepper

1. Cook the Brussels sprouts in salted boiling water for 5 minutes, until nearly tender. Add the peas, return to a boil, and cook for 2 minutes, then drain and place in a serving dish.
2. Meanwhile, melt the butter or spread in a small pan. Add the hazelnuts and cook for 1 minute, until golden. Add the orange zest and juice and cook for 1 minute.
3. Season with salt and pepper and pour over the sprouts and peas to serve.

Peperonata

I adore ratatouille in the late summer months and serve it with fish, poultry, and also as a stand-alone dish. Peperonata is along similar lines, made with colorful bell peppers and tomatoes, and can be prepared well in advance of eating and serving. I like to serve it with roast chicken and spicy sausages, but it's also good served cold as part of an antipasti. Any leftovers will also be welcome with pasta or as an omelet filling. It also freezes well, so it's worth making in bulk.

○ ○ ●	SERVES 4	V	✱
PER PORTION:	CALORIES **120**	PROTEIN **4.3 g**	CARBOHYDRATE **22.6 g**	FAT **1.3 g**

Low-fat cooking spray

2 red onions, peeled and thinly sliced

2 garlic cloves, crushed

2 bay leaves

4 red bell peppers, seeded and thinly sliced

2 yellow bell peppers, seeded and thinly sliced

One 14-ounce (400 g) can diced tomatoes

Salt and freshly ground black pepper

2 tablespoons chopped fresh basil

1. Generously spray a large nonstick pan with low-fat cooking spray. Heat, add the onions, garlic, and bay leaves, and cook gently for 5 minutes, stirring occasionally.
2. Add the bell peppers, tomatoes, and salt and pepper, mixing well. Cook, uncovered, for about 20 minutes, stirring occasionally. Discard the bay leaves.
3. Stir in the basil and serve warm, or let cool and then chill until ready to serve.

Zesty Lemon and Chive Hummus

A spoonful of hummus makes a flavorful mouthful at almost any stage after WLS, but it's especially welcome the moment you can tolerate soft foods. Much later, it becomes a great standby as a dip, a side dish for roasted meats, a topping for a baked potato, or a sandwich spread instead of butter. I also like to thin it a little and use as a dressing for bean and grain salads. It's a cinch to make in the blender or food processor and tastes so much better homemade than many of the commercial offerings.

	SERVES 4		Ⓥ
PER PORTION:	CALORIES 115	PROTEIN 5.8 g	CARBOHYDRATE 9.1 g	FAT 6.2 g

One 14-ounce (400 g) can chickpeas

2 tablespoons tahini paste

1 garlic clove, crushed

Grated zest of 1 lemon

Juice of 2 lemons

Salt and freshly ground black pepper

1 tablespoon snipped fresh chives

1. Drain the chickpeas, rinse them in cold water, and drain again thoroughly.
2. Place them in a blender or food processor with the tahini, garlic, lemon zest, lemon juice, and season with salt and pepper. Blend on high power to make a smooth purée.
3. Fold in the snipped chives, then spoon into a small serving dish. Cover and chill until ready to serve.

Guacamole

Guacamole is the perfect healthy dip for vegetable crudités, so there is always some in my refrigerator. It is also superb as a buffet-table side dish, but a scoop is also very welcome with a one-pot chili when feeding a crowd. I often add a scoop to the top of a baked potato, but love to add a spoonful to a breakfast omelet with some diced tomatoes and a sprinkling of cheese. It does have fat, but trust me, it's the good kind!

○ ● ●		SERVES 4		Ⓥ
PER PORTION:	CALORIES **78**	PROTEIN **1 g**	CARBOHYDRATE **2.4 g**	FAT **7.2 g**

1 ripe avocado

½ small red onion, very finely chopped

2 tomatoes, finely chopped

Juice of ½ lime

Salt and freshly ground black pepper

1 tablespoon chopped fresh cilantro, to serve

1. Peel the avocado, remove the pit, and mash the flesh coarsely.
2. Add the onion, tomatoes, lime juice, and salt and pepper. Add half the cilantro and mix well.
3. Spoon into a serving dish and sprinkle with the remaining cilantro.

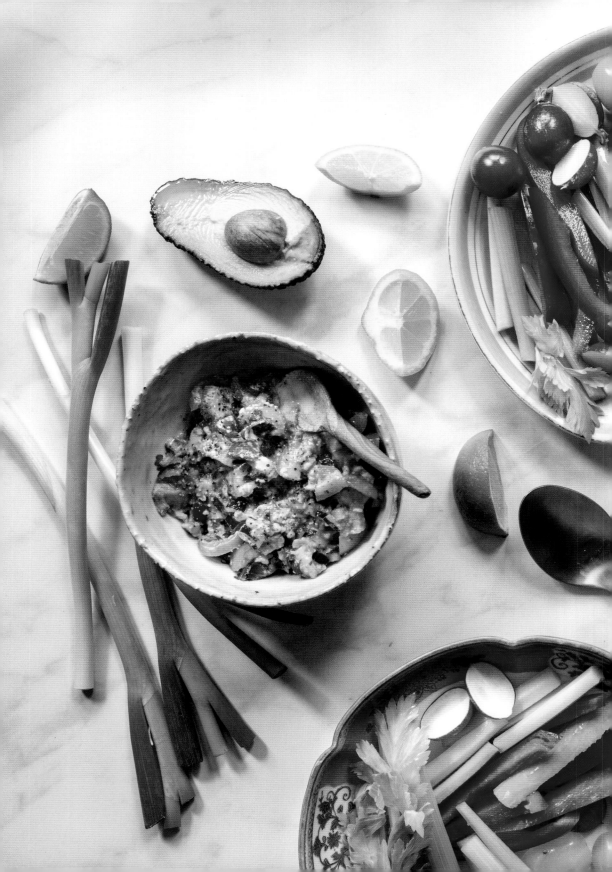

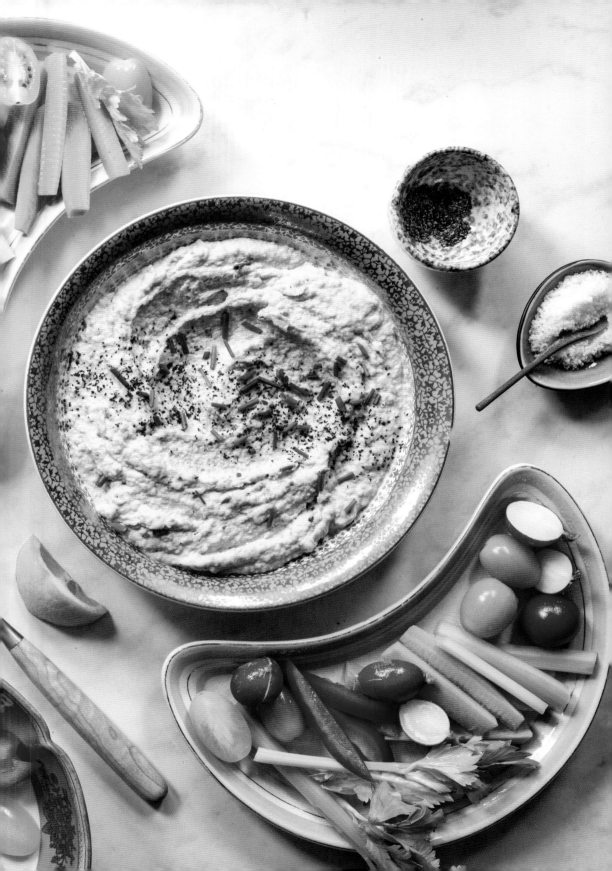

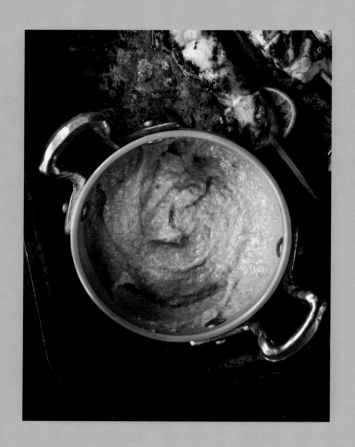

Dressings
and Sauces

———

Ranch Salad Dressing

WLS PORTION: ½–1

A very good salad can be ruined by a poor store-bought dressing, and it's one item I almost always make from scratch. Many ready-made dressings are full of sugars, use inferior seasonings, and are off the scale when it comes to salt, fat, and preservatives. So here is a very simple one to make that is also extremely versatile. It's flavorful and creamy and only has about 15 calories per serving. Use it for salads, as a dip, or in dishes where dressing or mayonnaise is required.

	MAKES ABOUT **15** PORTIONS		**V**
PER PORTION:	CALORIES **15**	PROTEIN **0.6 g**	CARBOHYDRATE **2 g**	FAT **0.5 g**

Generous ²/₃ cup (160 ml) skim milk

2 teaspoons white wine vinegar

Generous ²/₃ cup (160 ml) extra-light mayonnaise

½ teaspoon garlic powder

¼ teaspoon onion powder

1 teaspoon mustard powder

1 teaspoon chopped fresh parsley

4 scallions, finely chopped or ¼ cup (5 g) snipped
    fresh chives

Salt and freshly ground black pepper

1. Mix the milk with the vinegar in a bowl and allow to stand for 10 minutes.
2. Whisk the milk mixture with the mayonnaise, and the garlic, onion, and mustard powders, until smooth.
3. Add the parsley, scallions, and salt and pepper. Cover and chill, to thicken slightly. The dressing will improve and become more flavorful as it keeps.

Minty Yogurt Sauce

WLS PORTION:
1–2 TBSP

This deceptively simple sauce has great flavor and complements all kinds of roasted and fresh vegetables. You can also use it as a dip, or thin it slightly with water, milk, or stock to make a salad dressing. I use whole-milk yogurt instead of Greek-style to make this sauce, and I find it gives the best results.

	MAKES 600 ml / 1 pint / 2½ cups ABOUT 8 SERVINGS	V

PER PORTION:	CALORIES 92	PROTEIN 2.6 g	CARBOHYDRATE 2.4 g	FAT 7.9 g

2 cups (450 g) whole-milk plain yogurt
¼ cup (50 ml) extra virgin olive oil
½ cup (15 g) finely chopped fresh mint
1 teaspoon grated lemon zest
1 tablespoon lemon juice
Salt and freshly ground black pepper

1. Mix the yogurt with the oil, mint, lemon zest, lemon juice, and season with salt and pepper, blending well. If you are preparing in advance, do not add the mint until about an hour before serving.

2. Cover and chill before serving. Refrigerate leftovers and use within 2 days.

Simple Shallot Satay Sauce

This super satay sauce is the perfect go-to dip for chicken skewers (see page 150), but it's also great with vegetable tempura—or as a dressing or sauce for noodles, if you can tolerate them. I used a tikka masala paste in the recipe below, but any ready-made curry paste would work just as well.

○ ◐ ●		SERVES 8		Ⓥ
PER PORTION:	CALORIES **102**	PROTEIN **2.1 g**	CARBOHYDRATE **2.9 g**	FAT **9.1 g**

2 teaspoons sesame oil, or other oil of your choice

3 shallots, roughly chopped

1 tablespoon curry paste

3 tablespoons smooth no-added-sugar peanut butter

5 ounces (160 g) coconut cream

Juice of 1 lime

1. Heat the oil in a small pan, add the shallots, and cook gently for 3 to 5 minutes, until they soften.
2. Stir in the curry paste, peanut butter, coconut cream, and lime juice, mixing well.
3. Bring to a simmer and cook for 5 to 8 minutes until the sauce has thickened, then blend with an immersion blender until smooth.
4. Serve warm with chicken skewers, vegetable tempura, or as a sauce for noodles or spiralized vegetables.

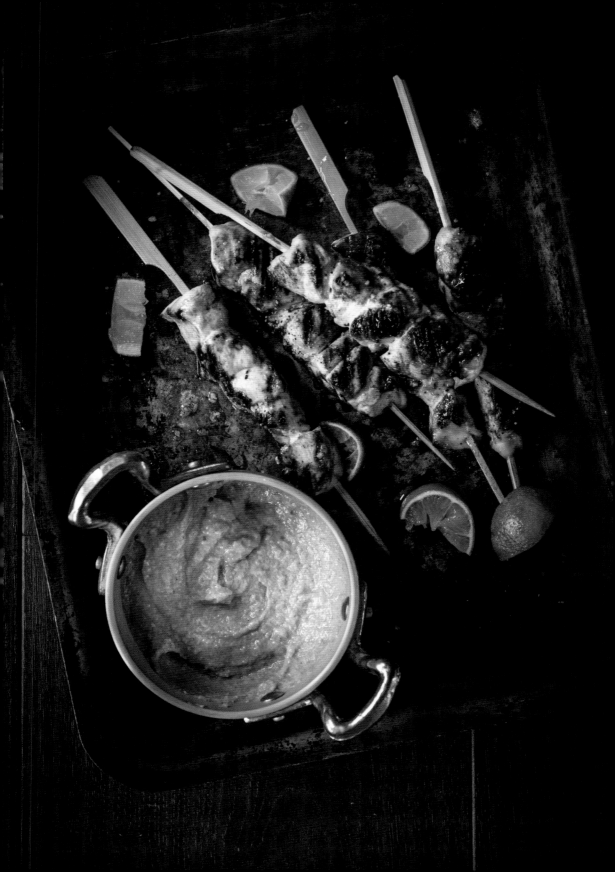

Tonnato Sauce

This is a thick, creamy tuna sauce which goes fantastically well over cooked chicken or turkey to make a classic Italian dish. I think it also makes a great dip or sauce for cooked or crisp vegetable crudités. If using for the former, decorate the finished dish in traditional style with sliced green olives and capers.

		SERVES 6		
PER PORTION:	CALORIES **93**	PROTEIN **9.1 g**	CARBOHYDRATE **2.9 g**	FAT **4.9 g**

8 ounces (225 g) tuna in oil, drained (reserve 1 tablespoon oil)

3 anchovy fillets

¾ cup (175 ml) light mayonnaise

2 teaspoons Dijon mustard

1 tablespoon lemon juice

Salt and freshly ground black pepper

1. Place the tuna and the reserved oil in a food processor or blender with the anchovies, mayonnaise, mustard, lemon juice, 1 tablespoon water, and season with salt and pepper. Blend until smooth.
2. Check the consistency of the mixture. It should be like a custard sauce—if necessary, add an additional tablespoon water and blend again.
3. Use to coat cooked and sliced chicken or turkey, or as a dip or sauce for cooked or crisp vegetables.

Egg Custard Sauce

WLS PORTION: ½–1

I frequently recommend a custard sauce for the early Soft Food (Yellow) stages, since it has some good protein and is gentle on the digestion. Ready-made canned varieties are available, but they are often either low in fat or low in sugar—rarely both. This one is much better. I make it with a semi-skim milk since I think the result is better with a milk slightly higher in fat. This nutritious custard is wonderful with mashed or sliced soft bananas or puréed fruit at the Soft Food (Yellow) stage, after quite some time on fluids only.

○ ◐ ●		SERVES 4		Ⓥ
PER PORTION:	CALORIES **132**	PROTEIN **7.5 g**	CARBOHYDRATE **9 g**	FAT **7.1 g**

2½ cups (600 ml) semi-skim or low-fat milk

4 large egg yolks

¼ cup (50 g) granulated sweetener

½ teaspoon vanilla extract

1. Pour the milk into a heavy pan and bring slowly to a boil.
2. In a large bowl, whisk the egg yolks with the sweetener and vanilla, until creamy.
3. Slowly pour the hot milk into the egg yolk mixture and whisk well to blend. Rinse out the saucepan.
4. Strain the mixture through a sieve back into the pan and place over low heat. Cook, stirring constantly, until the custard thickens enough to coat the back of a spoon and has the consistency of thick cream.
5. Serve plain, warm or cold, dusted with grated nutmeg, if desired, or with slices of banana or puréed fruit.

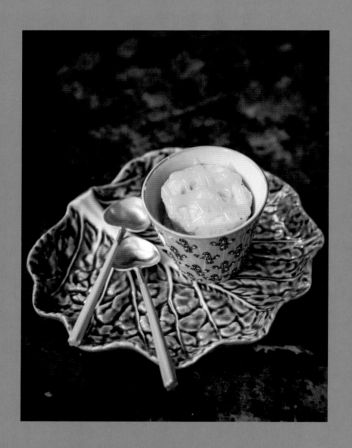

Desserts

—

Berry Compote with Whipped Ricotta

Here's a very simple dessert that looks impressive on the plate. Mixed berries are spooned onto whipped vanilla ricotta and sprinkled with crushed graham cracker crumbs. Decorate with a few sprigs of fresh herbs for a dazzling finale to a meal.

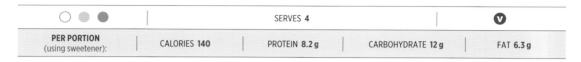

	SERVES 4		V
PER PORTION (using sweetener):	CALORIES **140**	PROTEIN **8.2 g**	CARBOHYDRATE **12 g**	FAT **6.3 g**

1¼ cups (200 g) blackberries

1¼ cups (200 g) raspberries

Sweetener, to taste, or 1 tablespoon confectioners' sugar

8 ounces (250 g) ricotta

1 teaspoon vanilla extract

2 graham crackers, crushed

Lemon thyme or mint sprigs, to decorate

1. Halve the blackberries if large and place in a bowl with the raspberries, sweetener to taste, and 1 tablespoon water. Stir well to crush very slightly, and let stand while preparing the ricotta.
2. Put the ricotta and vanilla in a food processor and blend until smooth and creamy.
3. Divide the ricotta between serving plates, spreading with the back of a spoon. Pile the fruits on top with their syrup.
4. Scatter with the crushed graham cracker crumbs and decorate with a few sprigs of fresh herbs to serve.

Cheesecake with Fig, Orange, and Ginger Topping

WLS PORTION: ½

This cheesecake looks divine and tastes even better, yet takes only minutes to prepare. I have served it here with a fig and ginger topping but you can serve it with almost any fresh fruit in season—berries, sliced citrus fruits, or a medley.

○ ○ ●		SERVES 8		V		✳
PER PORTION (without topping):	CALORIES **254**	PROTEIN **12.6 g**	CARBOHYDRATE **26.8 g**		FAT **10.9 g**	

¼ cup (50 g) butter

2½ tablespoons (50 g) honey

1²⁄₃ cups (150 g) oats

1¾ cups (400 g) low-fat cream cheese, softened

3 eggs, separated

¼ cup plus 2 tablespoons (75 g) granulated sweetener

1 teaspoon vanilla extract

4 ripe figs

2 oranges, peeled, pith removed, and sliced crosswise

2 tablespoons no-added-sugar apricot jam

2 tablespoons ginger wine, warmed

1. Preheat the oven to 350°F (180°C).
2. Melt the butter and honey in a pan and then stir in the oats, mixing well. Press into the bottom of an 8-inch (20 cm) nonstick springform cake pan.
3. Whisk the cream cheese with the egg yolks, sweetener, and vanilla, until smooth.
4. Whisk the egg whites until stiff, then fold into the cream cheese mixture. Pour onto the cheesecake crust.
5. Bake for 35 to 40 minutes, or until golden and just firm to the touch. Let cool before removing from the pan and transferring to a serving plate.
6. Cut the figs into thin slices and place them on top of the cheesecake, overlapping them in a circular pattern with the orange slices. Mix the apricot jam with the ginger wine to make a glaze, and brush over the figs. Chill to serve.

Quick Chocolate Mousse

This has to be the simplest and quickest chocolate mousse recipe I know. All you need are 2 ingredients—chocolate and eggs. The chocolate can be any kind you like and can tolerate—I have tested this with unsweetened chocolate, diabetic and protein chocolate, and all types from milk to white and dark, plus flavored chocolates. I find somewhere in the middle, between unsweetened and sweetened milk chocolate, is about right for me (and I like an orange-flavored one), but you'll know your own likes and dislikes. The recipe below is for 4 regular servings using unsweetened chocolate but all you need to remember is that you need 1 ounce (25 g) chocolate and 1 egg for a regular serving (about 2 WLS servings). The mixture can also be flavored with grated orange zest or chopped ginger. Serve topped with a little low-fat whipped topping or yogurt, if desired, and decorated with fruit in season. Easy-peasy, but looks like a million dollars!

○ ● ●	SERVES 4	Ⓥ

PER PORTION (using unsweetened chocolate):	CALORIES **182**	PROTEIN **8.1 g**	CARBOHYDRATE **13.5 g**	FAT **12.6 g**

4 ounces (100 g) chocolate, broken up

4 eggs, separated

1. Melt the chocolate in a bowl over boiling water, or in the microwave, and let cool, until barely warm.
2. Add the egg yolks to the chocolate and mix well.
3. Whisk the egg whites in a clean bowl until they stand in stiff peaks. Fold into the chocolate mixture with a metal spoon. Spoon into glasses and chill to set, about 2 to 3 hours.

Protein Ice Cream

It can be hard in the early days after surgery to meet your daily protein requirement, but I found one of the easiest ways was to make a protein ice cream with a flavored whey protein powder. There are a vast number of protein powders out there to experiment with and you'll find the ones you like. I found some very sweet and some granular, but what suits one won't suit all. Use this simple recipe as the basis for experimenting further—you can always add unsweetened chocolate pieces, chopped nuts, and fruit to the mix. Plus you can make it thicker and richer by using fat-free yogurt for half of the milk. Play with the flavors and prepare to be surprised.

● ● ●	SERVES 4	Ⓥ	✳
PER PORTION (using milk and typical protein powder):	CALORIES **133**	PROTEIN **27.2 g**	CARBOHYDRATE **6.3 g**	FAT **0.1 g**

2¼ cups (500 ml) low-fat milk, or milk and yogurt combined

Four 1-ounce (27 g) scoops low-fat and low-sugar vanilla whey protein isolate powder

1. Mix the milk with the protein powder in a large bowl, beating well to combine.
2. Pour into an ice cream maker and process until softly whipped and frozen. Spoon into one large or four small freezer containers and freeze until firm. You could also serve it softly frozen at this stage, if you prefer. Alternatively, pour into a large freezer container and freeze until firm, whisking once or twice during the freezing process to break down any large ice crystals.
3. Remove from the freezer 30 to 60 minutes before serving to soften slightly for scooping.

VARIATIONS

Chocolate: Use 4 scoops chocolate protein powder with 2 tablespoons unsweetened cocoa powder and a few squares of chopped unsweetened chocolate, if desired.

Frappuccino: Use 2 scoops chocolate and 2 scoops coffee protein powder.

Frozen Yogurt Fruit Layer Cake

This is a stunning sweet treat of a dessert—layered stripes of fruit and yogurt that is simply sliced or cut into wedges to serve. It can be made in a loaf or round cake pan and decorated with seasonal fruits, mint leaves, and edible flowers for a grand finale.

○ ● ●	SERVES 6		Ⅴ	✳
PER PORTION:	CALORIES **105**	PROTEIN **9 g**	CARBOHYDRATE **16.5 g**	FAT **0.4 g**

8 ounces (250 g) frozen mixed berries

1 pound (450 g) fat-free plain Greek yogurt

2 tablespoons granulated sweetener

8 ounces (250 g) mango, chopped

11 ounces (300 g) kiwi fruit, chopped

Fresh fruit, mint leaves, and edible flowers,
   to decorate (optional)

1. Put a quarter of the frozen berries on the bottom of a 9 x 5-inch (23 x 13 cm) loaf or 9-inch (23 cm) round cake pan.
2. Blend the remainder of the berries with 6 ounces (150 g) of the yogurt and 1 tablespoon of the sweetener. Spread over the berries in the pan and freeze for 1½ hours.
3. Blend the mango with 7 ounces (200 g) of the yogurt and spread over the berry layer. Freeze for another 1 hour, until solid.
4. Blend the kiwi with the remaining yogurt and sweetener and spread over the mango layer. Cover with plastic wrap and freeze for 2 hours.
5. To serve, turn out onto a plate, wait 15 minutes to allow the cake to soften, then slice to serve, decorated with fresh fruit, mint leaves, and edible flowers, if desired.

Heavenly Coffee Ricotta Parfait

WLS
PORTION:
½–1

I first made this deceptively simple dessert on a day when all seemed to go wrong (and all the more miserable-making because it was so wonderfully bright, warm, and sunny). It was heavenly . . . hence the name!

○ ● ●		SERVES 1		**V**		**✳**
PER PORTION:	CALORIES **170**	PROTEIN **11.8 g**	CARBOHYDRATE **3.7 g**	FAT **11.9 g**

4 ounces (125 g) ricotta
1 teaspoon instant coffee
Granulated sweetener, to taste
A few chocolate coffee beans, to serve (optional)

1. Mix the ricotta with the coffee and sweetener until smooth. Spoon into a plastic-wrap–lined small bowl and level the surface. Cover again with plastic wrap and then freeze until firm, at least 2 hours.
2. To serve, carefully unwrap the ricotta parfait and turn out onto a serving plate, removing and discarding the plastic wrap. Top with a few chocolate coffee beans, if desired.

Raspberry Fro-Yo

Here's a healthier alternative to full-fat, sugary ice cream. It's great for all occasions—in a dish with fruit, in a cone, or frozen on a stick, popsicle style. You can serve it immediately, or freeze in an airtight container (but bring out of the freezer and let it stand for about fifteen minutes to soften, so that scooping is easier).

○ ◐ ●	SERVES 6	Ⓥ	✳
PER PORTION:	CALORIES **115**	PROTEIN **11.3 g**	CARBOHYDRATE **9.4 g**	FAT **3.5 g**

3 cups (350 g) fresh or frozen raspberries
2 cups (500 g) fat-free plain Greek yogurt
7 ounces (200 g) unsweetened condensed milk

1. If using fresh raspberries, place them in a container and freeze until solid. Once solid, put them in a food processor and blend until finely chopped. Remove 3 to 4 tablespoons and reserve for serving with the fro-yo. If using frozen berries, finely chop and reserve some in the same way.
2. Add the yogurt and condensed milk to the food processor and blend until everything is combined. The raspberries will have frozen the other ingredients to make a soft-scoop textured ice. Serve immediately or turn into a freezer container and freeze until firm.
3. Serve scoops of the fro-yo topped with a sprinkling of the reserved raspberry bits.
4. If serving later, remove from the freezer about 15 minutes before serving, so it's easier to scoop.

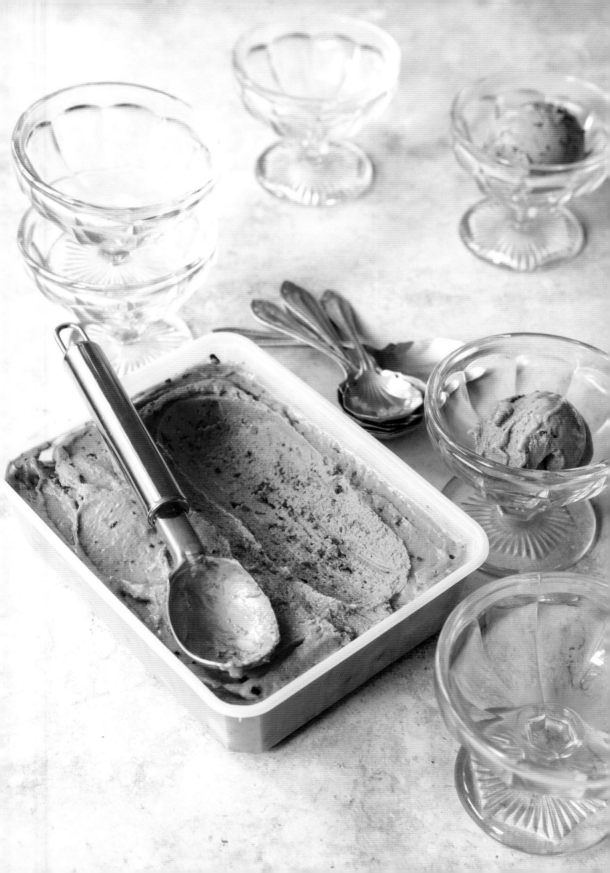

Zesty Lemon Curd Cake Cups

Nothing could be simpler than adding a few ingredients to a cup or mug and zapping it in the microwave to produce a warm, steamed, sponge-like cake ready for instant eating. This lemon one is especially good and is best eaten warm, straight from the cup—it does tend to lose all its appeal and lusciousness if left to cool and firm. It's a once-in-a-while sweet dessert when nothing else will do.

○ ◐ ●	MAKES 2	Ⓥ

PER PORTION:	CALORIES 340	PROTEIN 9.1 g	CARBOHYDRATE 35 g	FAT 18.2 g

¼ cup plus 2 tablespoons (48 g) all-purpose flour

½ teaspoon baking powder

Pinch of salt

1 egg, beaten

Grated zest of ¼ lemon

2 tablespoons granulated sweetener or sugar

2 tablespoons vegetable oil

¼ cup plus 2 tablespoons (90 ml) low-fat milk

2 teaspoons lemon curd

1. Put the flour, baking powder, salt, egg, lemon zest, sweetener, oil, and milk in a bowl and stir well until smooth. Divide between 2 large microwave-safe mugs or cups (with about ⅔ cup/150 ml capacity).
2. Cook in the microwave for 2 minutes.
3. Let cool for a few minutes. The cakes will shrink away from the sides of the cup. Top with the lemon curd.
4. Serve while still warm and eat from the cup.

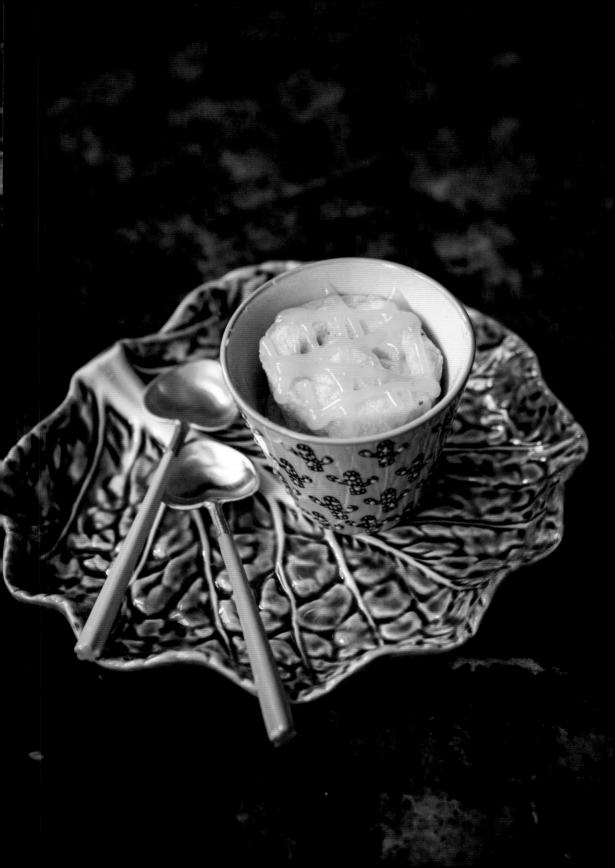

Toffee Apple Bariatric Crumble

Spoons at the ready! Here's a dessert that few can resist. Made with an apple, cinnamon, and orange base, it is finished with a great bariatric-friendly topping of oats and almonds with vanilla protein powder. Change your sweetener to honey, maple syrup, or artificial sweetener, if preferred.

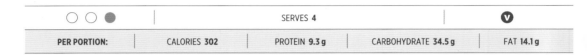

		SERVES 4		V
PER PORTION:	CALORIES **302**	PROTEIN **9.3 g**	CARBOHYDRATE **34.5 g**	FAT **14.1 g**

3 large apples, peeled, cored, and chopped

1½ teaspoons low-sugar fruit syrup

¼ teaspoon ground cinnamon

½ teaspoon coconut oil or melted low-fat spread

Juice of ½ small orange

For the Protein Crumble Topping

1 ounce (25 g) vanilla protein powder

1 cup (100 g) oats

¼ cup (25 g) ground almonds

2 tablespoons coconut oil or melted low-fat spread

1½ teaspoons low-sugar fruit syrup

1. Preheat the oven to 325°F (170°C).
2. Place the apples, syrup, cinnamon, coconut oil, and orange juice in a large pan and cook, until the liquid starts to caramelize and the apples soften. Spoon into a baking dish.
3. Meanwhile, mix the protein powder with the oats and ground almonds. Add the coconut oil and rub together with the fingertips to make a light crumble topping. Sprinkle on top of the apple base.
4. Bake until the crumble topping is lightly browned—this may only take about 5 minutes, and check frequently because it can color very quickly.
5. Serve warm with low-fat and reduced-sugar custard, yogurt, or low-fat ice cream, as desired and tolerated.

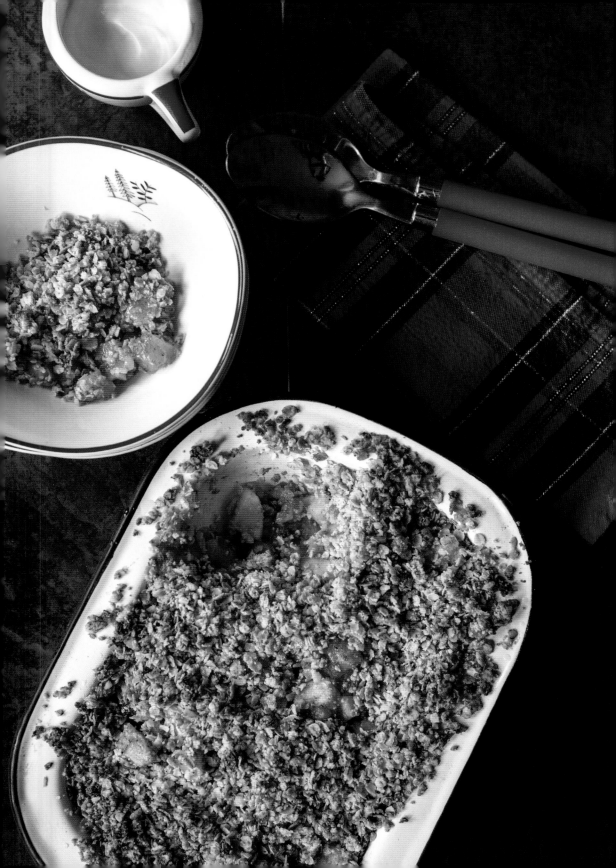

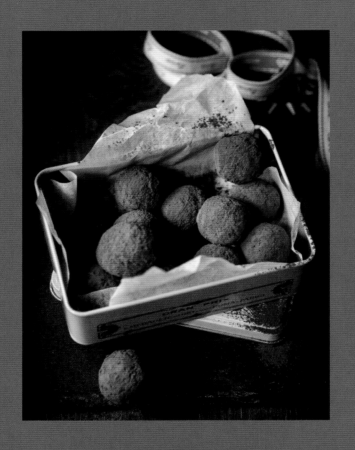

Snacks
and Treats

—

Healthy Peanut Butter Apple Slices

Apple slices make a great snack when reserves are running low, and when loaded with peanut butter, celery, raisins, and a few pumpkin seeds, they are highly nutritious.

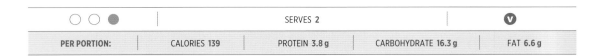

○ ○ ●		SERVES 2		**V**
PER PORTION:	CALORIES **139**	PROTEIN **3.8 g**	CARBOHYDRATE **16.3 g**	FAT **6.6 g**

1 apple

1½ tablespoons reduced-fat and no-added-sugar peanut butter

½ stalk celery, thinly sliced

1 tablespoon raisins

1 tablespoon pumpkin seeds

1. Core and slice the apple into rings.
2. Spread each slice with the peanut butter and top with the celery.
3. Dot with the raisins and sprinkle with the pumpkin seeds to serve.

Avocado and Bacon Deviled Eggs

WLS PORTION: 1

My refrigerator is rarely without a few hard-boiled eggs, since they make easy snacking with the bonus of great protein. I use them for lunch with salad, too. They also make great appetizers for handing around at parties or other gatherings—I simply mash the cooked yolk with a little yogurt or light mayonnaise, and seasonings like herbs, curry powder, and unusual spices. Here's an idea that takes the humble stuffed egg to a new level!

	MAKES 12		
PER EGG HALF:	CALORIES 75	PROTEIN 5.7 g	CARBOHYDRATE 0.9 g	FAT 5.5 g

6 large hard-boiled eggs, peeled

3 tablespoons low-fat mayonnaise

2 teaspoons Dijon mustard

1 tablespoon finely snipped chives or scallions

1 small avocado, peeled and mashed roughly with a fork

3 slices lean cooked bacon, crumbled

Salt and freshly ground black pepper

1. Slice the eggs in half lengthwise and scoop out the yolks into a small bowl, reserving the egg-white halves.
2. Add the mayonnaise, mustard, half of the chives, avocado, most of the bacon, and season with salt and pepper, then mash, mixing well.
3. Spoon evenly into the egg whites, and place on a serving plate.
4. Sprinkle with the remaining chives and bacon. Cover and chill until ready to serve.

Versatile Smoked Salmon Pâté

Pâté is another food I tend to stockpile in my fridge or freezer because it lends itself to a speedy lunch, great starter, or necessary snack. A few slices of cucumber or a crisp protein-based cracker topped with a little pâté settles and abates the cravings. This smoked salmon one can be adapted for other smoked fish, like trout or mackerel, and you can make it in a thrifty way by purchasing trimmings, rather than the more expensive slices or fillets.

			SERVES 6		
PER PORTION:	CALORIES **60**	PROTEIN **9 g**	CARBOHYDRATE **1.5 g**	FAT **2 g**

5 ounces (150 g) smoked salmon slices, or smoked salmon trimmings

5 ounces (150 g) quark

½ teaspoon finely grated lemon zest

1 tablespoon lemon juice

2 teaspoons prepared horseradish

A few drops of Tabasco sauce

2 teaspoons snipped fresh chives

1. Place the salmon, quark, lemon zest, lemon juice, horseradish, and Tabasco in a food processor or blender, and blend to a smooth, creamy paste.
2. Spoon into a jar or serving dish, then cover and chill until ready to serve. The pâté will keep in the refrigerator for 3 to 4 days.
3. Serve sprinkled with snipped chives.

Snack Attack Microwave Chips

WLS PORTION: ½–1

I never encourage anyone to snack or graze, but in an imperfect world, I do recognize that there are times when you want a crispy fix. My advice here is to stay clear of the fat-laden, ready-made options. As tempting as they might be with their "lower-fat, high-protein, calorie-reduced" promises—they rarely are a healthy option. Instead, why not make these microwave vegetable chips? You can experiment and vary the flavorings with jerk seasoning, curry and chili powder, and dried herbs, as desired.

A WORD OF CAUTION: These are made on a plate suitable for microwave cooking, but it may discolor with prolonged or repeated use, so use an old one rather than your best china to prepare these crunchy lifesavers.

○ ○ ●	SERVES 2			V
PER PORTION (for potatoes):	CALORIES 74	PROTEIN 1.8 g	CARBOHYDRATE 15.7 g	FAT 0.6 g

6 ounces (175 g) baking potato (or similar weight of raw root vegetables, such as parsnip, beet, celery root, or carrot)

Low-fat cooking spray

Seasonings to sprinkle, as desired, to serve

1. Very thinly slice the potato or other root vegetables (a mandoline is useful, though not essential to do this). Dry or remove any excess moisture with paper towels.

2. Generously spray a large microwave-safe plate with low-fat cooking spray. Spread the potatoes or vegetables in a single layer over the plate and spray again (you may have to do this in batches).

3. Microwave for 6 to 10 minutes, until golden and crispy. Times will depend on the power of your microwave but also the chosen vegetable—check frequently.

4. Remove from the plate and sprinkle with seasonings to serve. Store in an airtight container.

Spicy Roasted Chickpeas

These are the perfect replacement for nuts or other crunchy snacks post-op. They are best served warm but can obviously be eaten cold. Play around with the seasonings to find a combination you really like—the cumin and smoked paprika one here is just a starting point.

		SERVES 4		V
PER PORTION:	CALORIES **79**	PROTEIN **4.7 g**	CARBOHYDRATE **10.3 g**	FAT **2.1 g**

14-ounce (400 g) can chickpeas, drained and rinsed

1 teaspoon ground cumin

1 teaspoon smoked paprika

Cayenne pepper (optional)

Salt and freshly ground black pepper

Low-fat cooking spray

1. Preheat the oven to 350°F (180°C).
2. Pat dry the chickpeas with paper towels, and spread out on a nonstick baking sheet.
3. Sprinkle with the cumin, paprika, cayenne pepper to taste, if using, and season with salt and pepper. Spray with low-fat cooking spray until well-coated.
4. Roast for 25 minutes, shake to turn over, and roast for an additional 20 minutes. Serve warm, or allow to cool and store in an airtight container until ready to serve.

Passion Fruit and Pomegranate Bark

WLS PORTION: ½–1

This is one of those little treats that tastes far, far better than the sum of its individual parts, and is so very easy to make. Plain Greek yogurt is mixed with a little sweetener, cornstarch, and fruit, and then topped with more fruit and frozen until firm. The result is a "bark" that can then be broken into pieces for easy eating. Just take from the freezer what you need and store the remainder for up to two weeks. If you don't tolerate fruit seeds too well, substitute with berries or other chopped fruit.

○ ○ ●	SERVES 6		Ⓥ	✳
PER PORTION:	CALORIES 52	PROTEIN 8 g	CARBOHYDRATE 4.9 g	FAT 0 g

1¾ cups (450 g) fat-free plain Greek yogurt

1 teaspoon cornstarch

1 tablespoon granulated sweetener of your choice

Pulp of 1 passion fruit

3 tablespoons pomegranate seeds

1. Mix the yogurt with the cornstarch and sweetener until well combined.
2. Stir through half the passion fruit and pomegranate seeds.
3. Turn onto a baking sheet lined with foil and spread as thinly or thickly as you like your bark to be.
4. Top with the remaining fruit, sprinkling evenly.
5. Freeze for about 1 hour, or until completely frozen.
6. To serve, remove from the freezer and use a sharp knife to break the bark into bite-size pieces. Freeze any leftovers in ziplock bags for up to 2 weeks.

Coconut Fruity Ice Pops

WLS
PORTION:
1

Sadly, there is little hope that a supermarket freezer or ice cream truck will have a low-fat, low-sugar, and supremely bariatric-friendly popsicle, so why not make your own? These are wonderful for those early post-op days when you hanker after something cooling and not just water, and ideal for those summer days when you're further along your diet and fancy a fruity treat. If you don't have popsicle molds, you can use disposable plastic cups and wooden sticks instead.

	MAKES 8		V	✳
PER PORTION:	CALORIES **40**	PROTEIN **0.6 g**	CARBOHYDRATE **9.6 g**	FAT **0.1 g**

2½ cups (600 ml) unsweetened coconut water

1¼ pounds (600 g) cubed or sliced soft fruit (such as strawberries, mango, kiwi, or raspberries)

2 to 3 tablespoons agave nectar or your favorite sweetener

1. Place the coconut water and half of your chosen fruit in a blender, and blend until smooth. Add the agave nectar and blend again, adjusting the sweetness to taste (remember, sweetness diminishes with freezing).

2. Divide the remaining fruit among popsicle molds (about 8) then top with the puréed fruit mixture.

3. Freeze for at least 4 hours, or overnight, until solid.

4. To remove the popsicles from the molds easily, try plunging them briefly in warm water to tease them out.

NOTE: If you are at the early onset of the full Liquid (Red) or Soft Food (Yellow) stage, feel free to purée the entire recipe to a suitable texture and consistency before freezing, rather than leaving the fruit whole.

VARIATION If you don't like coconut, use low-fat yogurt instead.

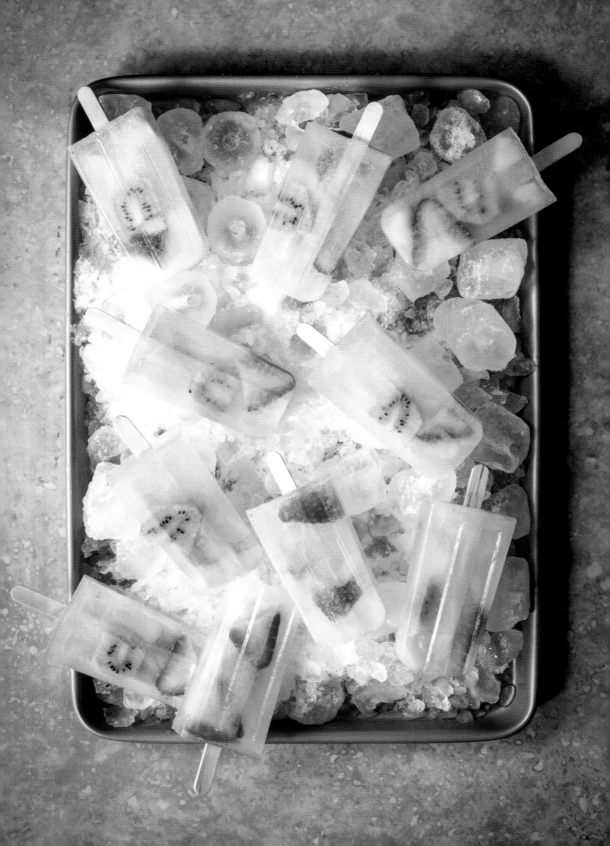

Fruit, Nut, and Chocolate Bites

WLS
PORTION:
1

I first made these little "truffle" bites for Easter as an allowable chocolate treat, again at Christmas, and I make them every now and again because they are gorgeous. So much better than "energy balls" and the healthy treats on the shelves in supermarkets. Don't forget to soak the nuts ahead of time—this reduces the need to add oil.

○ ○ ●		MAKES 20		V
PER PORTION (without whole nut decoration):	CALORIES **49**	PROTEIN **1.6 g**	CARBOHYDRATE **4.6 g**	FAT **2.9 g**

1 cup (100 g) mixed broken nuts, soaked in water
   for 8 hours
4 ounces (100 g) soft pitted prunes
4 ounces (100 g) soft dried apricots
2 tablespoons unsweetened cocoa powder
Extra cocoa powder, to dust
20 whole nuts, to decorate (optional)

1. Drain the nuts and place in a food processor with the prunes and apricots. Pulse until they are well broken up and have formed a soft doughy mixture that holds together.
2. Remove and stir in the cocoa powder—it will take a little time, but will mix in. Divide and roll into about 20 balls.
3. Coat each with a little extra cocoa powder. Stud the top of each with a whole nut, if you wish.

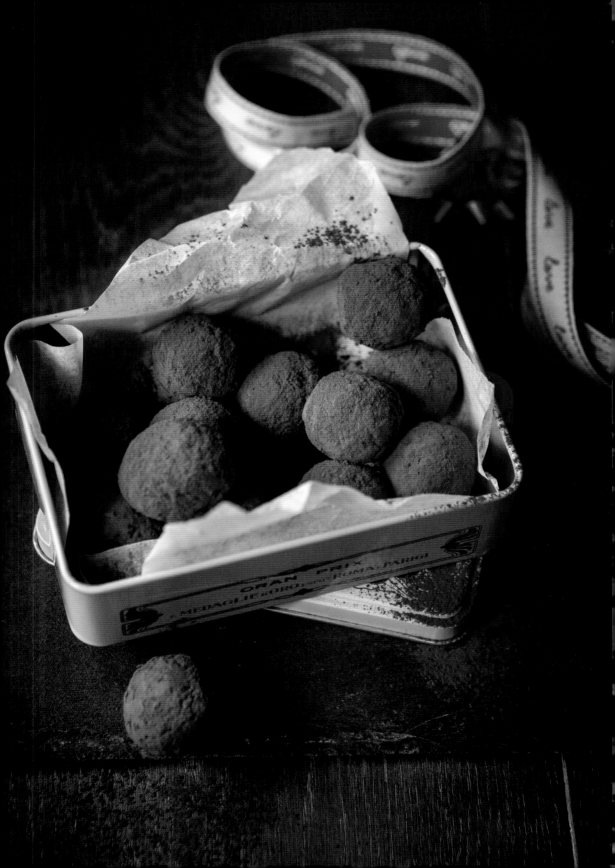

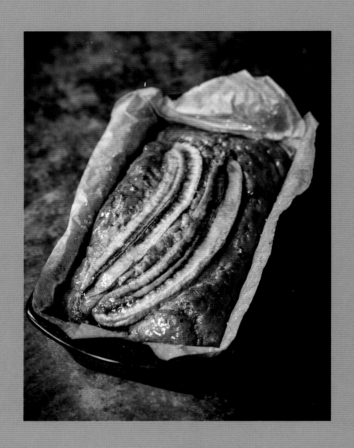

The Great Bariatric Bake-Off

—

Protein Loaf

Many bariatric patients struggle to eat bread in the early days (and sometimes later) but hanker for a slice of something. This useful and versatile loaf might be the answer. It's a high-protein, gluten-free, freezable loaf that can be eaten sweet or savory. It makes a great sandwich, and is fabulous as a side to soup, wonderful toasted, and just the thing to eat as an afternoon treat with bariatric-friendly jam. It's also ideal for those who want a low-carb alternative.

	MAKES **1** LARGE LOAF (about **16** slices)	**V**

PER PORTION (using butter and no topping):	CALORIES **152**	PROTEIN **7.2 g**	CARBOHYDRATE **2.7 g**	FAT **12.3 g**

2 cups (200 g) ground almonds or almond flour

¼ cup plus 2 tablespoons (42 g) coconut flour

1½ teaspoons baking powder

Scant ½ teaspoon baking soda

Large pinch of salt

7 large eggs

3 tablespoons melted butter or coconut oil

1 heaping tablespoon honey

1½ tablespoons apple cider vinegar

Golden flaxseeds or chopped nuts, to sprinkle (optional)

1. Preheat the oven to 375°F (190°C). Grease a large loaf pan (about 8½ inches long/22 cm).
2. Mix the ground almonds with the coconut flour, baking powder, baking soda, and salt in a bowl.
3. In a second bowl, beat the eggs with the butter, honey, and vinegar.
4. Pour the egg mixture over the dry ingredients and whisk until smooth and combined.
5. Transfer to the loaf pan, smooth the top and sprinkle with the flaxseeds, if using. Bake for 35 to 40 minutes, until golden and shrinking from the sides of the pan.
6. Run a knife around the edges of the pan and turn out onto a wire rack to cool. Serve sliced.

Peanut Cookies

WLS PORTION: 1

It's hard to come up with a cookie recipe that isn't high in sugar, calories, and fat, but this one does score well on paper and plate. I have used a one-for-one sweetener—if yours doesn't replace sugar in this ratio, then adjust accordingly. Store in an airtight container for up to three days—if they last that long!

	MAKES 24		V

PER COOKIE:	CALORIES 107	PROTEIN 3.5 g	CARBOHYDRATE 8.9 g	FAT 6.4 g

6 tablespoons (75 g) light butter, or reduced-fat margarine, softened

8 ounces (225 g) no-added-sugar crunchy peanut butter

1 large egg, beaten

2 tablespoons honey

½ teaspoon vanilla extract

1 ounce (25 g) granulated sweetener

2 cups (200 g) all-purpose flour

½ teaspoon baking powder

1. Preheat the oven to 350°F (180°C). Line 2 large baking sheets with parchment paper.
2. In a large bowl, whisk together the butter or margarine with the peanut butter until well combined.
3. Beat in the egg, honey, vanilla, and sweetener.
4. Sift the flour with the baking powder, add to the peanut mixture, and beat until well combined.
5. Take 24 walnut-sized balls of the mixture and place on the lined baking sheets, about ¾ inch (2 cm) apart. Flatten slightly with the tines of a fork.
6. Bake for 8 to 10 minutes, or until golden and set. Cool on a wire rack until cold, then store in an airtight container for up to 3 days.

Best-Ever Bariatric Brownies

I have made a few variations of brownies over the years, but these truly have to be the best. I'm happy to serve them plain in all their squidgy glory, but for a special treat, they can be topped with a cocoa-flavored cream cheese or Quark-flavored frosting (and a mini candied egg for Easter, perhaps).

○ ○ ●		MAKES **9** SQUARES/**6** MUFFIN ROUNDS		**V**
PER SQUARE/ROUND:	CALORIES **54/81**	PROTEIN **4.7 g/7.1 g**	CARBOHYDRATE **8.2 g/12.2 g**	FAT **1.8 g/2.7 g**

Low-fat cooking spray

6½ ounces (185 g) fat-free plain Greek yogurt

3 tablespoons low-fat milk

½ cup (45 g) unsweetened cocoa powder

½ cup (40 g) rolled oats

6 tablespoons granulated sweetener

3 tablespoons unsweetened applesauce or purée

1 egg, beaten

2 teaspoons baking powder

Pinch of salt

1. Preheat the oven to 400°F (200°C). Spray a 6-inch (15 cm) square shallow cake pan, or a 6-cup muffin pan, with low-fat cooking spray. Line the pan with parchment paper, if desired, for easy release. The former will provide a cake that can be cut into 9 squares; the latter, 6 deeper muffin rounds (with a slightly more squidgy center).

2. In a large bowl, mix the yogurt with the milk, cocoa, oats, sweetener, applesauce, egg, baking powder, and salt, beating well to combine.

3. Spoon the mixture into the pan, or divide evenly between the muffin cups and level the surface. Bake in the cake pan for 20 to 25 minutes, or the muffin pan for 18 to 20 minutes, until firm on top but still slightly sticky in the middle. Remove from the oven and allow to cool in the pan.

4. Slice the square cake into 9 pieces to serve, or unmold the round brownies to serve whole.

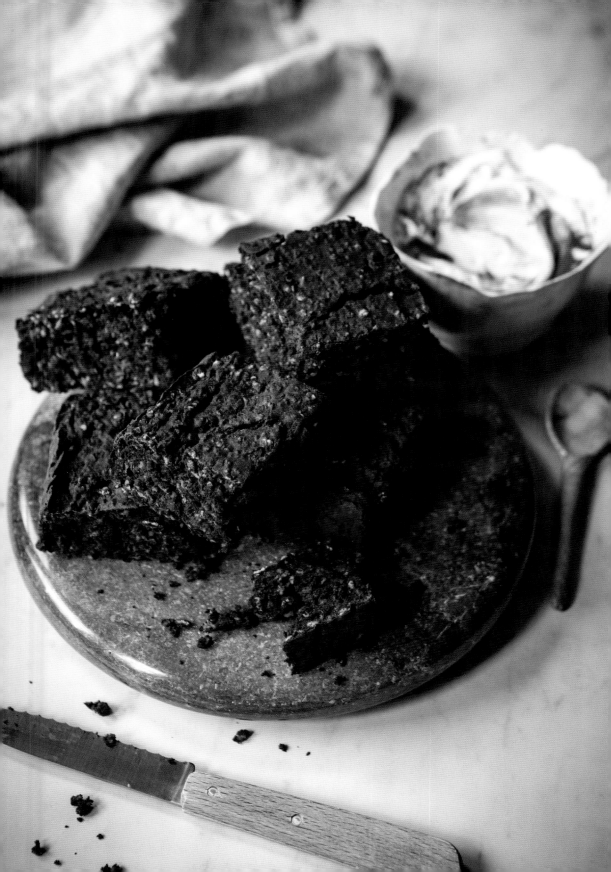

Apple and Blackberry Cake

This is a favorite cake recipe that I make every year when we've been blackberry picking. It only needs a handful to supplement the apples, but they are all the better for being in the mix. It's good hot, warm, and cold; served sliced plain, or with custard, yogurt, or low-fat ice cream.

○ ○ ●		SERVES 8		Ⓥ
PER PORTION:	CALORIES **175**	PROTEIN **5.9 g**	CARBOHYDRATE **21.4 g**	FAT **7.3 g**

1 cup (100 g) all-purpose flour

1 heaping tablespoon granulated sweetener

2 teaspoons finely grated lemon zest

2 teaspoons baking powder

3 eggs

3 tablespoons low-fat milk

3 ounces (75 g) low-fat spread or light butter, melted

2 pounds (900 g) assorted apples, peeled, cored, and cut into slices

Low-fat cooking spray

½ cup (100 g) blackberries

2 tablespoons sliced almonds

Sifted confectioners' sugar, to decorate (optional)

1. Preheat the oven to 400°F (200°C).
2. In a large bowl, mix the flour with the sweetener, lemon zest, and baking powder. Make a well in the center and add the eggs and milk. Whisk, then add the melted spread or light butter and mix well.
3. Add the apple slices to the batter and fold in lightly.
4. Spray a 9-inch (23 cm) nonstick springform pan with low-fat cooking spray. Add the batter and sprinkle with the blackberries and sliced almonds. Bake for 30 to 40 minutes, until well-risen, firm, and golden.
5. Allow to cool slightly before serving, dusted with confectioners' sugar, if desired. Cut into slices to serve.

Zesty Clementine Cake

Here's a cake that I make in the winter months when citrus fruits are at their best, cheapest, and most plentiful. Indeed, it has taken over from our Christmas cake on a couple of occasions, since it can be prettied up with fruit slices on the top. It's a moist cake that isn't overly sweet and keeps fresh for several days. It's heavier than a traditional sponge, but not too dense for the bariatric to digest. It is also lovely served with light cream, yogurt, or custard.

○ ○ ●		SERVES 12		Ⓥ
PER PORTION:	CALORIES **270**	PROTEIN **9.1 g**	CARBOHYDRATE **14.7 g**	FAT **19.8 g**

14 ounces (400 g) whole clementines, with skin

Low-fat cooking spray

Scant ½ cup (125 g) honey

3 tablespoons olive oil

5 eggs

3 cups (300 g) ground almonds or almond flour

1½ teaspoons baking powder

1. Place the clementines in a pan, and cover with water. Weight down with a smaller pan lid so that the clementines stay submerged in the water. Bring to a boil, lower the heat, and cook for 45 to 60 minutes, until they are very tender. Drain and let cool. When cool, cut in half and remove any seeds.

2. Preheat the oven to 350°F (180°C). Line the bottom of a 8½-inch (22 cm) springform pan with parchment paper and spray the sides with low-fat cooking spray.

3. Place the cooked clementines in a food processor and blend until smooth.

4. Add the honey, olive oil, and eggs, and pulse to combine.

5. Mix the ground almonds with the baking powder, add to the clementine mixture, and pulse until just mixed—do not overprocess. Pour the mixture into the prepared pan and bake for 50 minutes, or until the cake is well-risen, golden, firm to the touch, and a skewer inserted into the center of the cake comes out clean. Cover the top of the cake with foil or parchment paper if it starts to brown too much (check after 30 minutes).

6. Let cool in the pan, then turn out to serve, and cut into thin wedges. Decorate the top with a few slices of fresh clementine if serving on the same day. Use candied or dried clementine if storing for longer.

Farmhouse Banana Loaf

This is a tweak of a recipe that my grandmother used to make—a sort of light, fruited loaf stuffed with nuts and dried fruit. This isn't as loaded with fat or sugar as the original, due to the cunning use of bananas for moistness and sweetening power. I like to halve a banana lengthwise and pop it on top of the loaf before baking for an indulgent flourish.

○ ○ ●	MAKES 12 SLICES	Ⓥ	✳
PER SLICE (without additional topping):	CALORIES **135**	PROTEIN **3.5 g**	CARBOHYDRATE **21.7 g**	FAT **3.6 g**

Low-fat cooking spray

2 tablespoons low-fat spread or light butter

1 ounce (25 g) granulated sweetener

1 egg

2 large bananas, mashed

1½ cups (175 g) all-purpose flour

1½ teaspoons baking powder

1 teaspoon baking soda

1 teaspoon ground cinnamon

½ cup (50 g) mixed chopped nuts

Generous ½ cup (75 g) raisins

3 tablespoons low-fat milk

1 banana, peeled and halved lengthwise, to decorate (optional)

1. Preheat the oven to 350°F (180°C). Line an 8½ x 4½-inch (22 x 11½ cm) nonstick loaf pan with parchment paper and spray with low-fat cooking spray.

2. Beat the spread or butter with the sweetener until pale and light, then beat in the egg. Fold in the mashed bananas and mix well.

3. Mix the flour with the baking powder, baking soda, and cinnamon, and fold into the banana mixture.

4. Fold in the nuts, raisins, and milk, and mix well.

5. Spoon into the prepared pan and top with the banana halves, if using. Bake for 45 to 50 minutes, covering with a little foil for the last 5 minutes of cooking time if the loaf starts to brown too much. Allow to cool on a wire rack.

6. Slice to serve. Store in an airtight container for up to 3 days.

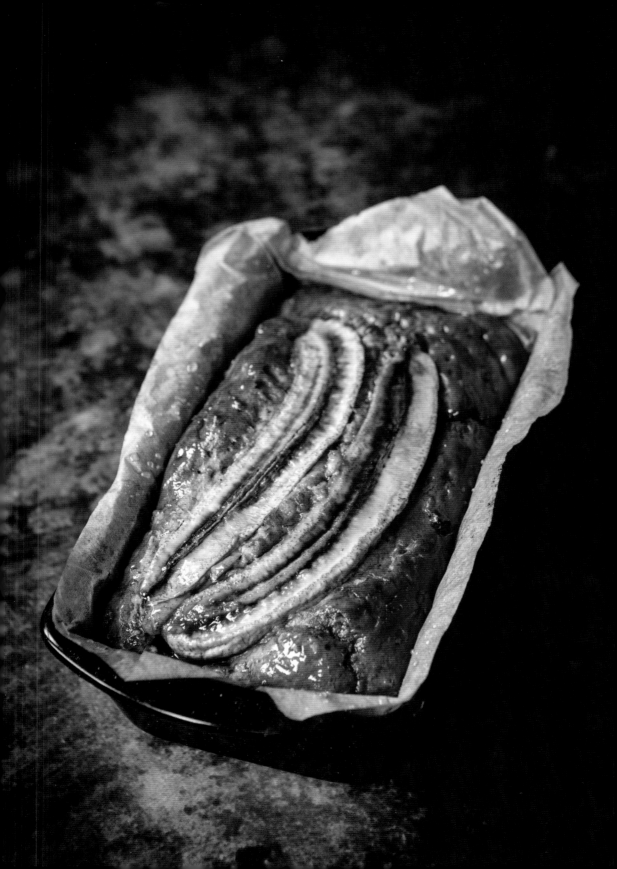

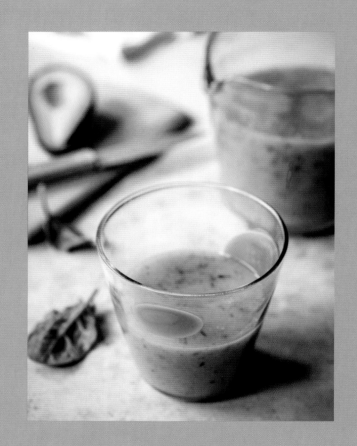

Drinks, Shakes, and Meals in a Glass

—

Frozen Berry Smoothie Yogurt Glass

Not everyone likes the taste or texture of protein powder, but most like the idea of a smoothie. This one doesn't use a protein powder but still provides a hefty dose of protein and can be made with frozen berries.

● ● ●		SERVES 1		Ⓥ
PER PORTION:	CALORIES **102**	PROTEIN **12.2 g**	CARBOHYDRATE **11 g**	FAT **0.4 g**

½ cup (100 g) high-protein vanilla yogurt

3 tablespoons low-fat milk

About 30 frozen mixed berries

1. Place the yogurt, milk, and berries in a blender or food processor and blend until smooth.
2. Pour into a glass and serve.

Icy Protein Mocha

I am amazed at how many post-ops turn to coffee as their new favorite drink after surgery. If you're one of them, you could do worse than to make this icy mocha drink rather than heading to the nearest coffee shop or drive-through.

● ● ●		SERVES 1		Ⓥ
PER PORTION:	CALORIES **114**	PROTEIN **15.4 g**	CARBOHYDRATE **5.6 g**	FAT **2.7 g**

1 shot espresso

2 tablespoons low-fat milk

1 ounce (25 g) low-fat and low-sugar chocolate or mocha protein powder

About 4 ice cubes

1. Place the coffee, milk, protein powder, and ice cubes in a blender or food processor, and blend until smooth.
2. Pour into a glass and serve.

Strawberry Dream Cream Shake

As the name suggests, this is a shake that tastes like strawberry ice cream—indulgent but compliant.

● ● ●		SERVES 1		Ⓥ
PER PORTION:	CALORIES **113**	PROTEIN **15.4 g**	CARBOHYDRATE **9.7 g**	FAT **1.5 g**

½ cup (100 g) low-fat plain cottage cheese

3 tablespoons low-fat milk

6 frozen strawberries

Granulated sweetener, to taste

1. Place the cottage cheese, milk, strawberries, and sweetener to taste in a blender or food processor and blend until smooth.
2. Pour into a glass to serve.

Pumpkin Pie Shake

Nothing represents autumn more than pumpkin pie, and although we have made a version for bariatrics as a treat, you can still get the taste and experience in a shake and with a protein boost, too. Drink it plain or go full-out with a special topping—a squirt of low-fat or fat-free whipped topping and a sprinkling of nuts, if you like.

● ● ●		SERVES 1		Ⓥ
PER PORTION (without optional topping):	CALORIES **154**	PROTEIN **22.8 g**	CARBOHYDRATE **4.3 g**	FAT **4.6 g**

1 ounce (30 g) vanilla whey protein powder of your choice

1 cup (250 ml) low-fat unsweetened nut milk

¼ teaspoon pumpkin pie spice (more if you like a stronger flavor)

¼ teaspoon ground cinnamon

Ice cubes

Low-fat whipped topping and sprinkling of chopped nuts, to decorate (optional)

1. Place the protein powder, milk, pumpkin pie spice, cinnamon, and a little ice in a blender or food processor, and blend until smooth and well-mixed.
2. Pour into a serving glass and top with a squirt of low-fat whipped topping and a sprinkling of chopped nuts to serve, if desired.

Five-a-Day Smoothie

I'm frequently asked if I can recommend a protein drink or smoothie for the first Fluid (Red) stage of "eating" after surgery. Many protein drinks are overly sweet and synthetic-tasting—so I preferred to stick to milk, soups, and smoothies during this short period of time. As for the smoothie, this recipe has become a "stayer," and I still have it now and then as a meal in a glass (often when I'm in a hurry in the morning). It's called Five-a-Day because it has the ideal daily dose of fruit and vegetables recommended for a healthy diet. Occasionally, I have added a scoop of flavorless or vanilla-flavored protein powder to boost the protein, but you could just as easily add some dried milk powder, too.

		SERVES 2		Ⓥ
PER PORTION:	CALORIES **283**	PROTEIN **3.2 g**	CARBOHYDRATE **40.8 g**	FAT **12.5 g**

1 apple

1 pear

Scant ½ ounce (10 g) spinach leaves

¼ cup plus 1 tablespoon (70 g) low-fat coconut milk

¼ ripe avocado, peeled, pitted, and chopped

⅔ cup (150 ml) fresh orange juice

1. Core the apple and pear and cut into small chunks.
2. Place in a blender, food processor, or smoothie maker with the spinach, coconut milk, avocado, and orange juice. Pulse until smooth.
3. Pour into a glass to serve.

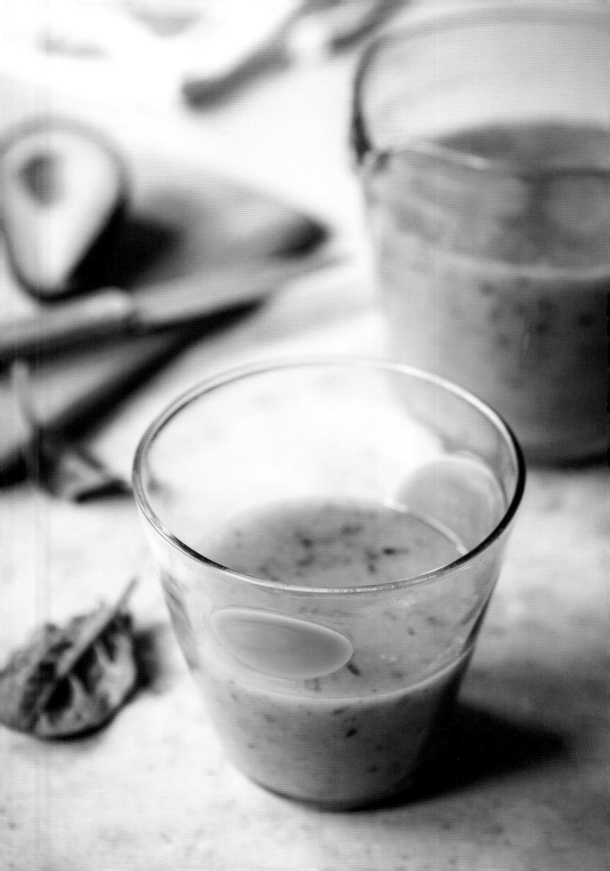

Winter Sunshine Smoothie

I hadn't thought too much of a smoothie for winter drinking until I was introduced to the benefits of turmeric. It combines well with coconut, ginger, clementines, and oats in this smoothie, a great internal engine boost for the darker months of the year.

	SERVES 2	V

PER PORTION:	CALORIES 192	PROTEIN 5.1 g	CARBOHYDRATE 40.8 g	FAT 2.1 g

⅓ cup (25 g) rolled oats

1 cup (225 ml) chilled unsweetened coconut water

2 tablespoons unsweetened coconut milk

2 clementines, peeled and segmented

½-inch (1 cm) piece peeled fresh turmeric or ½ teaspoon ground

½-inch (1 cm) piece peeled fresh ginger

1. Place the oats in a blender or food processor and blend to a powder.
2. Add the coconut water, coconut milk, clementines, turmeric, and ginger, and blend until smooth.
3. Pour into a glass to serve.

Mulled Blueberry Warmer

WLS PORTION: ½–1

This is a kind of mulled wine substitute (without the wine) that is ideal for bariatrics or non-drinkers. It's a tipple that's much more exciting than a dreary weak fruit punch. Cheers!

● ◐ ●		SERVES **4**		**V**
PER PORTION:	CALORIES **68**	PROTEIN **0.5 g**	CARBOHYDRATE **14.3 g**	FAT **0.3 g**

1¼ pint (750 ml) no-added-sugar blueberry juice drink

1 teaspoon honey

4 ounces (100 g) mixed fresh or frozen berries

¼ teaspoon ground cinnamon

Small piece peeled fresh ginger, sliced

1 star anise

2 cloves

2 cinnamon sticks

1. Place the blueberry drink, honey, berries, and cinnamon in a blender and blend until smooth.
2. Pour the mixture into a pan and add the ginger, star anise, cloves, and cinnamon sticks.
3. Warm through gently without boiling. Strain and serve warm.

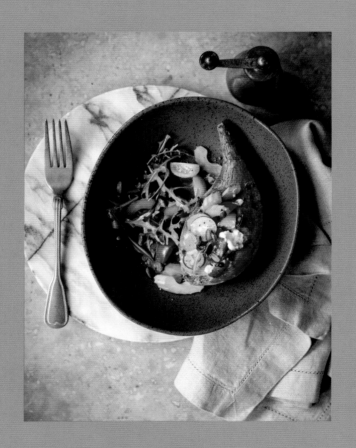

Solo Dining

—

Scrambled Egg in a Mug

WLS PORTION: 1

I make my Scrambled Egg in a Mug at least three times a week for breakfast, light lunch, or simply anytime. I don't tire of it because I add so many different things to mix it up. A few strips of cooked ham, slivers of smoked salmon, slices of mushrooms or peppers, a tablespoon of grated or crumbled cheese, a few snips of fresh herbs, or flakes of smoked fish bring variety. The secret to success is to add them just before you let the egg mixture stand—the residual heat will continue to cook the egg and warm the additions sufficiently enough for serving.

		SERVES 1		V
PER PORTION:	CALORIES **105**	PROTEIN **9.1 g**	CARBOHYDRATE **1.3 g**	FAT **7 g**

1 large egg
1 tablespoon skim or low-fat milk
Salt and freshly ground black pepper

1. Break the egg into a 1¼-cup (300 ml) microwave-safe mug (you can use a smaller one if you do not intend to add any extra filling). Add the milk and salt and pepper, beating well with a fork.
2. Place in the microwave and cook for 30 seconds. Remove and beat the egg with a fork. Return to the microwave and cook for an additional 10 seconds. Remove and beat again. If the egg is still very runny, cook for an additional 10 seconds, or until the egg is almost set but still runny in places.
3. Add any chosen additions and mix well. Let stand for 1 minute before serving with toast, if desired and tolerated.

Corn and Haddock Chowder in a Cup

WLS PORTION: 1

I made this hearty corn chowder with frozen smoked haddock but have since tried it with other types of fish (white fish, smoked fish, and shrimp) and it works equally as well. These seafoods are the kind of basic freezer staples to stash away for a meal when you are dining solo. It has an impressive amount of protein packed into the cupful. You can also stir in a handful of baby spinach leaves before leaving it to stand.

○ ● ● | SERVES 1

PER PORTION:	CALORIES 180	PROTEIN 19.7 g	CARBOHYDRATE 17.3 g	FAT 3.5 g

Low-fat cooking spray

2 teaspoons finely chopped onion

1 slice lean bacon, chopped

1 small potato, peeled and cut into small cubes

¼ cup (60 ml) skim or low-fat milk

2 tablespoons canned corn

3 tablespoons skinless smoked haddock pieces (defrosted, if frozen)

Freshly ground black pepper

Handful of baby spinach leaves (optional)

1. Generously spray the bottom of a 1¼-cup (300 ml) microwave-safe mug with low-fat cooking spray. Add the onion and bacon and microwave for 30 seconds.

2. Add the potato and ¼ cup (60 ml) water, mixing well. Microwave for 75 to 90 seconds, until the potato is almost tender.

3. Add the milk, corn, and haddock, and microwave for 45 seconds. Stir, taking care not to break up the fish too much, and microwave for an additional 30 to 40 seconds, or until the fish flakes easily and the potato is tender.

4. Season to taste with pepper, and add the spinach, if desired, mixing well. Let stand for 1 minute before serving.

Smoky Fish Frittata

Every now and again, there's a deal at my deli counter on a few slices of smoked salmon or a solitary peppered smoked mackerel or trout fillet that I know will make a good high-protein meal. Sometimes I use it to fill a wrap for a lunch box or flake it into a salad. Here's another way to use such versatile protein-packers for a main-meal dish that is quick and easy to prepare. It's also delicious served warm or cold.

	○ ○ ●		SERVES 1

PER PORTION:	CALORIES **240**	PROTEIN **26.9 g**	CARBOHYDRATE **2.1 g**	FAT **13.6 g**

2 eggs

3 tablespoons skim or low-fat milk

Salt and freshly ground black pepper

Low-fat cooking spray

2 ounces (50 g) hot smoked salmon or a small smoked fish fillet (peppered mackerel, kipper, or smoked trout), flaked or chopped

2 teaspoons snipped chives or 1 to 2 asparagus spears, cooked and chopped

1 teaspoon grated Parmesan cheese

1. Beat the eggs with the milk and salt and pepper until well-mixed. Preheat the broiler.
2. Generously spray a small nonstick omelet or sauté pan with low-fat cooking spray. Heat, add the egg mixture, and cook for 30 seconds.
3. Scatter over the flaked fish and chives or asparagus, and cook until the egg is almost set.
4. Sprinkle with the Parmesan cheese, place under the broiler, and cook until the cheese is golden. Serve at once, or allow to cool to serve.

Italian Meatballs in a Bowl

I think homemade meatballs are ridiculously easy to prepare at home—and then you know exactly what is in them. You can use any extra-lean ground meat you prefer, and season accordingly. I like to play around with chicken and turkey flavored with harissa; lamb Middle Eastern–style with cumin and cilantro; beef with dried herbs de Provence—and I am not averse to a vegetarian mixture. This Italian version uses lean beef and basil. When cooked with a tomato sauce, mixed vegetables, and stock, you get a kind of "stew" for one. When time is tight, you can use four small ready-made meatballs from the freezer—vegetarian, too, if preferred.

○ ○ ●		SERVES 1		
PER PORTION:	CALORIES **160**	PROTEIN **18.7 g**	CARBOHYDRATE **12 g**	FAT **4.2 g**

3 tablespoons lean ground beef

1 to 2 teaspoons chopped fresh basil

Salt and freshly ground black pepper

¼ cup plus 1 tablespoon (70 g) prepared tomato sauce or canned diced tomatoes with basil

¼ cup (60 ml) beef or chicken stock

2 tablespoons canned or frozen and defrosted mixed chopped vegetables

Chopped fresh basil, to garnish (optional)

1. **To make the meatballs,** mix the beef with the basil and salt and pepper. Divide and shape into 4 small balls.

2. Place the meatballs in the bottom of a small deep microwave-safe bowl (about 1¾ cups/400 ml). Cover and microwave for 1 minute. If using ready-made meatballs, halve this cooking time.

3. Stir in the tomato sauce, stock, mixed vegetables, and salt and pepper. Cover and microwave for 2 minutes. Stir, cover again, and microwave for an additional 1 minute, until hot and cooked through.

4. Let stand for 1 minute, then garnish with a little extra chopped fresh basil, if desired. Serve while still hot.

Chicken Waldorf Salad in a Jar

WLS PORTION: 1

One of my favorite salads pre-op was a Waldorf—classically made with lettuce, apple, celery, onion, walnuts, and grapes. I have now given it a bariatric makeover so that I can still enjoy it, since this one is lower in fat and higher in protein. How? By using Greek yogurt in the dressing and adding a little chicken for extra protein. The quantities in the recipe below make one jar for a bariatric-sized meal, but I often make two at a time and store in the fridge for up to five days. Placing the dressing in the bottom of the jar means you simply turn it upside down just before serving to mix the salad ingredients so that it doesn't get soggy. I turn it out onto a plate to serve but you can mix it in the jar, if taking it away from home as a portable or lunch box meal—just remember to take a fork.

				SERVES 1

PER PORTION:	CALORIES 197	PROTEIN 17.8 g	CARBOHYDRATE 16.4 g	FAT 7 g

2 tablespoons fat-free Greek yogurt, or plain low-fat yogurt

1 tablespoon extra-light mayonnaise

1 teaspoon snipped chives or 1 tablespoon grated cucumber

Juice of ½ lemon

Salt and freshly ground black pepper

1 stalk celery, chopped

¼ red onion, chopped

2 ounces (50 g) cooked skinless and boneless chicken, shredded or chopped (plain or seasoned)

2 walnut halves, roughly broken into pieces

½ apple, cored and chopped

3 grapes, halved

2 crisp lettuce leaves, shredded

1. **To make the dressing,** mix the yogurt with the mayonnaise, chives or cucumber, half of the lemon juice, and salt and pepper. If the yogurt is very thick, thin a little with some low-fat milk. Spoon into a small mason jar.

2. Top with the celery, then the red onion, chicken, walnuts, apple (tossed in the remaining lemon juice to prevent it from turning brown), grapes, and finally the lettuce. Cover with the lid and chill until ready to serve.

3. To serve, invert the jar so that the dressing drizzles through the salad mixture, or turn out onto a plate and toss lightly to mix.

Creamy Beany Chicken or Quorn

Using just four basic ingredients, this main-meal dish is the perfect one-pot meal for one. You can omit the crushed red pepper flakes if you don't like them, but they do add a little bit of zing without too much heat. I've used light cream, fat-free Greek yogurt, or quark in this recipe, and all work well to give a creamy result—but do be careful not to boil after adding, or the sauce might separate.

			SERVES 1			**V** (IF USING QUORN)

PER PORTION:	CALORIES **195**	PROTEIN **34.6 g**	CARBOHYDRATE **5.9 g**	FAT **3.4 g**

Low-fat cooking spray

1 small skinless and boneless chicken breast, sliced into thin strips, or 3 ounces (75 g) Quorn "chicken" pieces

2 ounces (50 g) French green beans, trimmed and halved if long

¼ teaspoon crushed red pepper flakes or ¼ teaspoon chile paste

4 to 6 cherry tomatoes, halved

3 tablespoons light cream, fat-free Greek yogurt, or low-fat quark

Salt and freshly ground black pepper

1. Generously spray a nonstick sauté pan with cooking spray. Heat, add the chicken strips or Quorn, and cook until opaque.
2. Add the green beans and crushed red pepper flakes and cook for 3 to 4 minutes, or until the beans are softened.
3. Add the tomatoes, mix well, and cook for 1 minute.
4. Stir in the cream, yogurt, or quark, season with salt and pepper, and reheat without boiling. Serve immediately.

Chicken Roast for One

This roast dish taxed my brain quite a bit in development—I didn't want to do the usual meat and vegetable but something easier instead. I like to think this works on a number of levels—it's not too time-consuming to make for one person (I fully understand that sometimes you just can't be bothered to cook for one), yet seems rewarding enough when cooked to justify the effort. It's a chicken breast roasted on a bed of creamy butternut squash with just a hint of chile to spice things up. I don't feel it needs anything extra, but you could serve with a green salad or a cooked green vegetable in season. Needless to say, the recipe serves one as a WLS portion.

○ ○ ● | SERVES 1

PER PORTION:	CALORIES **220**	PROTEIN **30 g**	CARBOHYDRATE **13.5 g**	FAT **5.3 g**

1 skinless and boneless chicken breast, about 3 1/2 ounces (100 g)

1/2 small red chile, finely chopped (according to taste)

A few sprigs fresh marjoram or oregano, chopped, or 1 teaspoon dried Mediterranean herbs

Salt and freshly ground black pepper

1/4 medium butternut squash, peeled, and seeded

1 tablespoon fat-free Greek yogurt or low-fat sour cream

Pinch of grated nutmeg

Low-fat cooking spray

1. Preheat the oven to 400°F (200°C).
2. Toss the chicken breast with the chile, herbs, and salt and pepper.
3. Slice the butternut squash as thinly as you can. Place a few slices in the bottom of a small roasting pan or dish that will snugly hold the squash and the chicken. Top with the remaining chicken and then fit the squash slices around it.
4. Carefully spoon the crème fraîche over the squash but not the chicken. Sprinkle with nutmeg and more salt and pepper to taste. Spray with cooking spray.
5. Roast for 25 to 35 minutes, or until the chicken is cooked and the squash is tender. Serve hot.

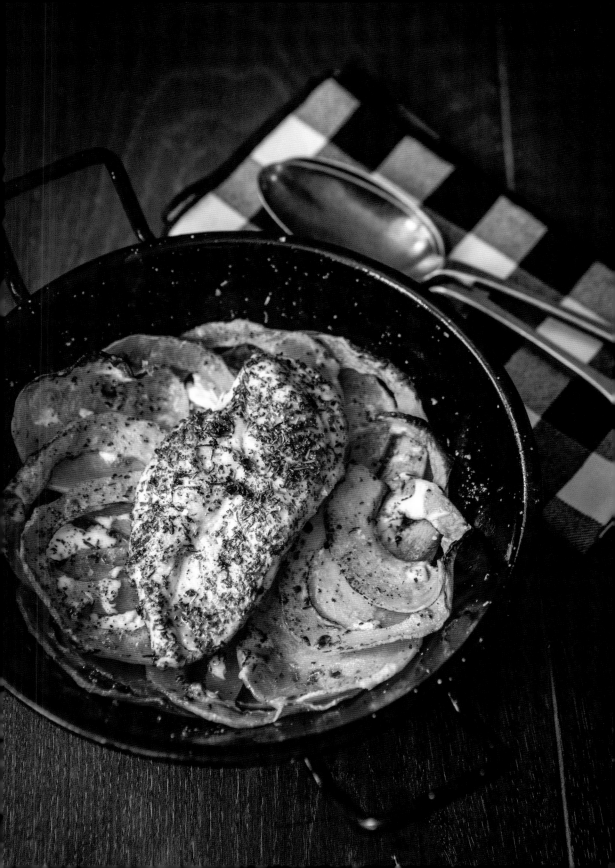

Baked Chicken Pesto

This is a dish I often make during the week, if dining alone. It's a simple four-ingredient dish that is easily prepared and quickly cooked. The small amount of pesto it uses lifts the chicken from the bland to the delicious. Serve with vegetables in season.

	SERVES 1			
PER PORTION:	CALORIES 248	PROTEIN 36.5 g	CARBOHYDRATE 4 g	FAT 9.8 g

1 skinless and boneless chicken breast, about
  4 ounces (115 g), flattened slightly

Heaping 1 teaspoon pesto sauce

Heaping 1 tablespoon grated or shredded reduced-
  fat mozzarella cheese

1 small tomato, sliced

1. Preheat the oven to 375°F (190°C).
2. Place the chicken on a small nonstick baking sheet and spread with the pesto sauce. Top with the cheese and the tomato. Cover with a little oiled foil and bake for 15 minutes.
3. Remove the foil and cook for an additional 5 to 10 minutes, or until the chicken is cooked through and no longer pink.
4. Serve with vegetables in season, if desired, or a crisp side salad.

Piquant Lamb Chops

This is one of the simplest dishes I know that is full of flavor and hits the spot every time. The flavors come from the tapenade (an olive and anchovy paste) and the tomato paste. I particularly like the one with sun-dried tomatoes in its mix. I splash out a little and buy the leanest, most tender French-style lamb cutlets for this recipe (you'll need two to three depending on size), but it works equally well with a rib chop. I don't think the chops need anything more than a salad or green vegetable accompaniment, but I often just have them on their own.

	SERVES 1		
PER PORTION:	CALORIES **185**	PROTEIN **30.5 g**	CARBOHYDRATE **1.2 g**	FAT **6.2 g**

1 lamb rib chop (about 1 pound/450 g)

1 teaspoon tapenade paste

1 teaspoon tomato paste

Finely chopped parsley and grated lemon zest, to serve (optional)

1. Preheat the broiler. Broil the rib chop under the grill, until any fat is golden and crisp and the lamb flesh is medium-rare.
2. Smear the meat with the tapenade and tomato paste and broil for an additional 30 seconds.
3. Sprinkle with parsley and lemon zest to serve, if desired.

Lighter Steak Stroganoff

I rarely feature a steak recipe for bariatric eating for three good reasons. First, beef or steak is usually only tolerated by a few, and then, only if chewed extensively (I think I am the exception). Second, it's pricey and so a real treat. And third, if you can afford and tolerate it, then, most often than not, you'll serve it simply cooked and won't need a recipe. But now and then, I come across a small steak that has been marked down in price and is just perfect for solo small-portion eating. Such a steak is also perfect for making into a stroganoff dish. Just a few sliced mushrooms and kitchen cupboard seasonings can make this already luxury dish a decadent one. Make it and savor every mouthful.

○ ○ ● | SERVES 1

PER PORTION:	CALORIES 225	PROTEIN 28.5 g	CARBOHYDRATE 12.7 g	FAT 5.2 g

Low-fat cooking spray

½ small onion, finely chopped

½ teaspoon garlic purée

¾ cup (75 g) sliced button mushrooms

Salt and freshly ground black pepper

3 ounces (75 g) lean beef steak (fillet or top round are good choices), cut into thin strips

2 teaspoons sherry or Madeira (optional)

1 teaspoon paprika

1 teaspoon Worcestershire sauce

1 teaspoon tomato paste

¾ teaspoon Dijon mustard

3 to 4 tablespoons quark

Chopped parsley, to garnish

1. Generously spray a nonstick sauté pan with cooking spray. Heat, add the onion, and cook for 4 minutes, until golden.
2. Add the garlic and mushrooms, then season well with salt and pepper. Cook over high heat for 4 minutes, or until the mushrooms are softened. Remove from the pan and keep warm.
3. Re-spray the pan, add the steak, and cook over high heat for 4 minutes, until just browned (do not overcook or the steak will toughen). Return the mushroom mixture to the pan with the sherry or Madeira, if using, and the paprika. Stir for 30 seconds.
4. Add the Worcestershire sauce, tomato paste, and mustard, and mix well.
5. Remove from the heat and stir in the quark. Gently reheat until the sauce is piping hot, but do not allow to boil. Serve immediately, sprinkled with parsley.

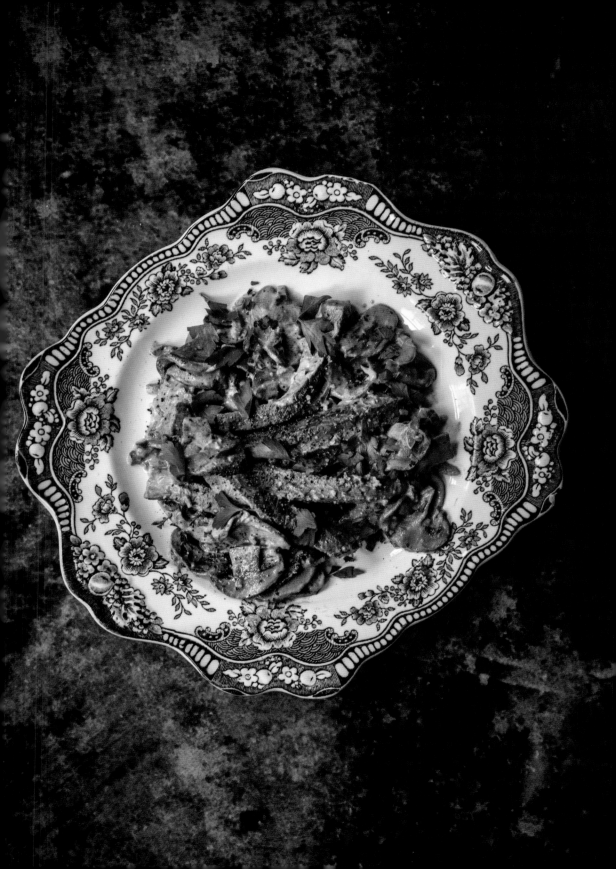

Ricotta, Celery, and Radish
Baked Sweet Potato

A simple mid-week meal, a baked sweet potato provides a great source of slow-release energy. Topped with light and creamy ricotta, crunchy vegetables, and seeds, this is a most healthy and satisfying meal for one.

○ ○ ●		SERVES 1		Ⓥ
PER PORTION:	CALORIES **215**	PROTEIN **7.1 g**	CARBOHYDRATE **34.6 g**	FAT **6.3 g**

1 small sweet potato

Low-fat cooking spray

1 tablespoon ricotta

Salt and freshly ground black pepper

½ stalk celery, sliced

3 radishes, sliced

2 cherry tomatoes, quartered

1 teaspoon pumpkin or sunflower seeds, toasted, if desired

1. Preheat the oven to 400°F (200°C). Scrub the sweet potato, prick in a couple of places, and spray lightly with cooking spray.
2. Bake for 30 to 40 minutes (depending upon the size), until tender. Remove and allow to cool slightly.
3. Meanwhile, season the ricotta with salt and pepper to taste.
4. Make a deep slit lengthwise along the sweet potato, open it out, and carefully mash the potato flesh with a fork. Top with the ricotta, celery, radishes, tomatoes, and seeds to serve.

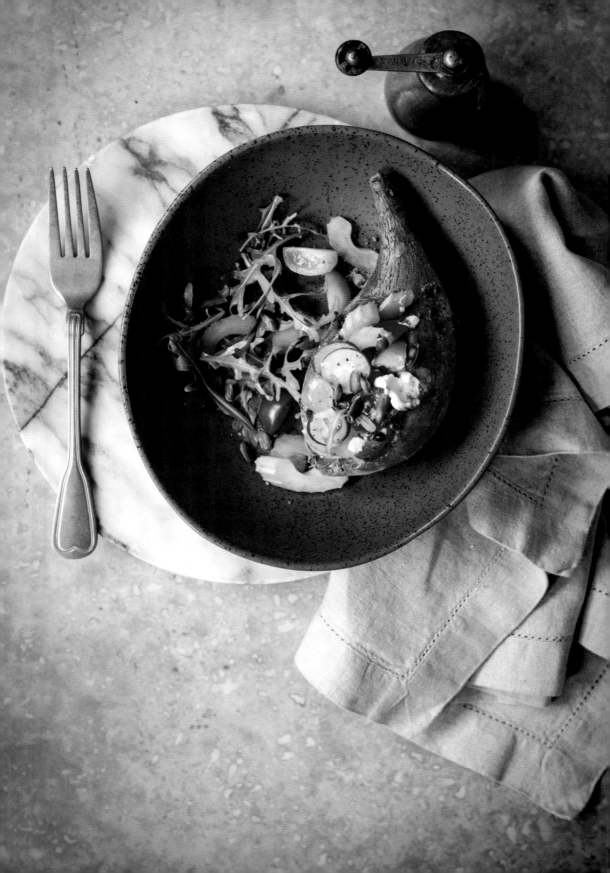

Easy Tiramisu for One

Over the years, I have developed many recipes for this wonderful coffee-flavored dessert, but this has to be the simplest one to date. It's perfect to make for solo eating. The secret is in using crispbread instead of sponge fingers, and a flavored quark mixture instead of cream. I have used a lemon one, but you can easily add lemon zest to a plain or vanilla-flavored one if you can't find it. It can be made up to a day ahead, but ideally needs about two hours chilling before serving. The recipe is for one, but can easily be doubled to serve two or more.

	SERVES 1		Ⓥ
PER PORTION:	CALORIES **142**	PROTEIN **10.6 g**	CARBOHYDRATE **21.4 g**	FAT **0.9 g**

1 crispbread (I use a high-fiber one)

1 to 2 tablespoons strong coffee (sweetened, if desired, with your chosen sweetener)

4 to 5 tablespoons lemon quark

Sweetener (optional)

Cocoa powder, to dust

1. Lightly crush or break the crispbread into pieces and place in the bottom of a small serving dish or ramekin. Spoon over the coffee.
2. Mix the lemon quark with sweetener to taste, if desired, and spoon over the crispbread base. Cover and chill for at least 2 hours.
3. Just before serving, dust the top with cocoa powder.

Very Berry Mug Crumble

This individual fruit crumble is a winner every time I make it—and because it uses mixed berries and autumn fruits from the freezer, it's a great standby recipe to round off a meal. If desired, you can substitute your favorite sweetener for the sugar, but there is only a little (unlikely to upset the WLS pouch or rock the scales) and it does help to give the crumble a bit of crunch.

○ ○ ●		SERVES 1		Ⓥ
PER PORTION:	CALORIES **180**	PROTEIN **3.4 g**	CARBOHYDRATE **34.2 g**	FAT **3.7 g**

About ½ cup (75 g) mixed frozen berries or sliced autumn fruit

½ to 1 teaspoon brown sugar

¾ teaspoon cornstarch

For the Crumble

3 tablespoons rolled oats

1½ teaspoons brown sugar

Pinch of ground cinnamon or ginger

1 teaspoon light butter or low-fat spread, melted

1. Place the frozen berries or autumn fruit in a small microwave-safe mug (about ¾ cup/ 125 ml)—they should almost fill the mug. Sprinkle over the sugar to taste and the cornstarch. Microwave for 30 seconds. Stir gently, trying to keep the fruit whole, then microwave for an additional 25 seconds, or until the sauces from the fruit start to thicken.

2. Meanwhile, for the crumble, place the oats in a small cup or bowl and stir in the sugar, cinnamon or ginger, and butter or spread. Mix well, then spoon over the partially cooked fruit mixture. Place the mug inside a shallow bowl (since the mixture does have a tendency to bubble over) and microwave for 75 seconds.

3. Let stand for 1 minute before serving with a little low-fat custard, yogurt, or low-fat ice cream, if desired.

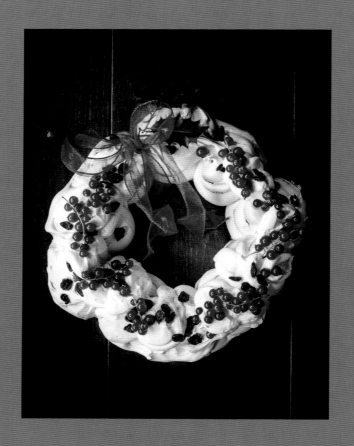

Holiday and Celebratory Specials

———

Party Appetizer Cups

I find preparing a bariatric-friendly antipasto feast is the way forward for party food—and if you gather and mix them together in a cup (with a handle for easy maneuvering) or small bowl, you will please WLS patients and others alike. Alternatively, provide empty cups with bowls of the foods suggested below so that guests can make their own selection. Either way, you'll find that everyone finds the WLS-friendly selection more to their liking rather than the usual greasy and beige offerings so often served at such gatherings.

TO CONSIDER

- **Protein:** An absolute and no-compromising must! Offer chunks of tuna, cubes of cooked meat and poultry, flakes or rolled-up pieces of smoked fish, cooked shrimp, slices of salami or other cooked and cured meats, and Quorn-style deli offerings.
- **Dairy:** Low- or reduced-fat mozzarella balls, cubes of low-fat cheese, pieces of feta cheese, halved or quartered hard-boiled small hen's or quail's eggs, quartered pieces of baby wax-coated cheeses, or mini peppers stuffed with light cream cheese.
- **Vegetables:** Chunks of cucumber, small cherry tomatoes, quartered canned artichoke hearts, roasted vegetables, and crisp vegetable sticks.
- **Legumes:** A drained and rinsed handful of chickpeas or giant lima beans.
- **Nuts:** A few roasted pine nuts, almonds, cashews, or peanuts will add a little crunch.
- **Seasoned seeds:** Sunflower, pumpkin, sesame, and flax—for more crunch with added nutrition.
- **Olives:** Green, black, stuffed, or exotically flavored—the choice is wide.
- **A little dressing** can be provided to moisten the combination. Choose your own low-fat version, or just a hummus mixture thinned with a little wine vinegar and a smidgen of oil.

Sweet Potato, Zucchini, and Cheese Mini Party Muffins

WLS PORTION:
1–2 (mini)
½–1 (large)

These little muffins are always popular at parties but also make small snacks for other times—as well as being a tasty lunch-box treat. The recipe will make thirty mini muffins or about fifteen larger ones.

○ ○ ●	MAKES **30** MINI MUFFINS/**15** LARGER MUFFINS	**V**	✱

PER MINI MUFFIN/LARGER MUFFIN:	CALORIES **38/76**	PROTEIN **2.5 g/5 g**	CARBOHYDRATE **2.9 g/5.8 g**	FAT **1.8 g/3.6 g**

Low-fat cooking spray

1 medium sweet potato, peeled and grated

1 red onion, very finely chopped or grated

1 medium zucchini, trimmed and grated

¼ cup plus 1 tablespoon (40 g) whole wheat flour

4 ounces (100 g) feta cheese, crumbled

½ cup (50 g) low-fat hard cheese, grated

4 eggs, beaten

Salt and freshly ground black pepper

1. Preheat the oven to 350°F (180°C). Spray mini muffin pans (ideally nonstick or silicone based) or large muffin cups with low-fat cooking spray, to prevent the muffins from sticking.
2. Mix the sweet potato with the onion, zucchini, flour, feta, hard cheese, eggs, and salt and pepper, mixing well.
3. Divide and spoon the mixture into the muffin cups—the mixture will make 30 mini muffins or about 15 larger ones.
4. Bake 15 minutes for the mini ones and about 20 to 22 minutes for the larger ones. Let cool and then turn out of the pans to serve.

Chicken Caesar Salad Cups

WLS PORTION: ½

Canapés and other party fare that are bariatric-friendly are often hard to find, so most patients end up eating the salad garnish! If you have the opportunity to take a dish to a party, consider this one—it's light and flavorful and can be enjoyed by one and all.

○ ○ ● | SERVES **6** (AS A STARTER OR MORE AS A CANAPÉ)

PER PORTION:	CALORIES **60**	PROTEIN **6.9 g**	CARBOHYDRATE **2.1 g**	FAT **2.5 g**

3 tablespoons extra-light mayonnaise

1 garlic clove, crushed

1 teaspoon Dijon mustard

2 tablespoons finely grated Parmesan cheese, plus a little extra to garnish

Salt and freshly ground black pepper

4 radishes, sliced

3 scallions, cut into thin strips

1 skinless and boneless cooked chicken breast, shredded

2 Little Gem lettuces

1. In a large bowl mix the mayonnaise with the garlic, mustard, Parmesan, and salt and pepper, beating well to blend.
2. Add the radishes, scallions, and chicken, and stir well to coat.
3. Separate the leaves of the lettuce and lay out on a serving plate. Spoon a little of the chicken mixture into each lettuce leaf. Sprinkle with a little extra grated Parmesan and chill to serve.

Red-Nose "Cupcake" Meatloaves

WLS PORTION: ½

These mini meatloaves have been a huge success every time I make them—so much so that I now frequently make half-size ones (baked in a mini muffin pan) for serving canapé-style at Christmas time. My original recipe here has a cauliflower mash "frosting" but it can easily be replaced for variety with virtually any other kind of mash, although the nutritional profile will change. They are a triumph because they can also be made well ahead and reheated easily.

○ ○ ● | SERVES **6** (**2 MEATLOAF CUPCAKES EACH**)

PER PORTION:	CALORIES **300**	PROTEIN **36.9 g**	CARBOHYDRATE **9.7 g**	FAT **6.8 g**

Low-fat cooking spray

2 pounds (900 g) extra-lean ground beef

1 cup (40 g) panko bread crumbs

2 egg whites, lightly beaten

2 teaspoons Worcestershire sauce

½ medium onion, very finely chopped

1 teaspoon steak seasoning or mixed dried herbs

Salt and freshly ground black pepper

1 medium head cauliflower

About 3 tablespoons fat-free plain Greek yogurt

12 cherry or grape tomatoes

Chopped fresh parsley, to garnish

Low-sugar ketchup, to serve (optional)

1. Preheat the oven to 375°F (190°C). Spray a 12-cup muffin pan with low-fat cooking spray.
2. Mix the ground beef with the bread crumbs, egg whites, Worcestershire sauce, onion, steak seasoning or herbs, and salt and pepper, mixing well. Divide into 12 portions and place in the prepared muffin cups. Bake for 20 minutes, until cooked through.
3. Meanwhile, trim and divide the cauliflower into florets and steam until soft. You can also cook them in the microwave (without additional water). Drain very well after cooking. Place in a food processor with the yogurt and salt and pepper, and purée until smooth.
4. To serve, spoon or pipe the cauliflower mash onto the top of each meatloaf, finish with a tomato "nose," and sprinkle with chopped parsley. Serve with a drizzle of ketchup or offer separately, if desired.

Salmon, Cucumber, and Avocado Timbales

This recipe has become quite a family favorite over the years, and I serve it as a starter at Christmas, Easter, and any celebration when I have a little time to cook on the same day. They can be made in advance, but not too far, as the avocado has a tendency to brown after a few hours.

○ ○ ●   SERVES **8**

PER PORTION:	CALORIES **190**	PROTEIN **20.7 g**	CARBOHYDRATE **4.6 g**	FAT **10.3 g**

Two 15-ounce (416 g) cans red or pink wild salmon, or about 1 pound (450 g) cooked fresh salmon

2 large tomatoes, seeded and finely chopped

1 large red onion, finely chopped

2 small ripe avocados, peeled, pitted, and finely chopped

¼ cucumber, seeded and finely chopped

¼ cup (15 g) chopped fresh cilantro

2 tablespoons lime or lemon juice

Salt and freshly ground black pepper

Salad greens, to serve

1. Drain the canned salmon, discarding the liquid. Remove any skin and bones, then break the flesh into small chunks. If using fresh salmon, flake the flesh into small chunks.

2. In a bowl, combine the tomato, onion, avocado, cucumber, cilantro, and lime or lemon juice. Add the salmon with salt and pepper to taste and mix gently.

3. Pack the mixture into 8 ramekins, or use metal rings, if you prefer. Cover and chill for at least 20 minutes, but do not prepare too far in advance or the avocado may turn brown.

4. Arrange salad greens on 8 serving plates, then turn out the timbales onto them to serve.

Yuletide Apple, Stilton, and Pecan Salad

WLS PORTION: ½

After the big festive Christmas or Thanksgiving feast, there are always turkey leftovers! Sometimes I make a curry or soup, but with the prime pieces that can still be carved, I serve this equally festive salad. It doesn't disappoint.

○ ○ ●		SERVES **4**		**V**
PER PORTION:	CALORIES **375**	PROTEIN **12.8 g**	CARBOHYDRATE **18.9 g**	FAT **27.3 g**

3 ounces (80 g) watercress or arugula, trimmed

5 ounces (150 g) baby spinach leaves

2 Pink Lady apples, cored and sliced

2 tablespoons lemon juice

2 stalks celery, thinly sliced

⅓ cup (50 g) golden or dark raisins

5 ounces (150 g) Stilton blue cheese, broken into chunks

¾ cup (75 g) pecans, broken into pieces

¼ cup (60 ml) fat-free dressing

½ teaspoon whole-grain mustard

1. Rinse and drain the watercress and spinach leaves thoroughly, then place on 1 large platter or 4 serving plates.
2. Toss the apple slices in the lemon juice and arrange on the salad greens with the celery, raisins, and Stilton cheese. Scatter the pecans over the top.
3. Mix the dressing with the mustard and drizzle over the salad mixture to serve.

Celebratory Spiced Salmon

Salmon—like turkey, ham, and other protein—makes a great centerpiece for a celebratory meal. Here, spices are used to great effect to cut through the richness of the flesh. The pomegranate molasses makes a great addition, but is optional if you are very sugar-sensitive. It is equally as good served hot or cold. Any leftovers can also be stir-fried with noodles for a quick and easy lunch dish.

		SERVES 8		
PER PORTION (without molasses):	CALORIES **212**	PROTEIN **26.8 g**	CARBOHYDRATE **0.9 g**	FAT **11.1 g**

2 to 2¼ pounds (900 g to 1 kg) whole side of salmon, trimmed and all bones removed

2 teaspoons sumac

1 teaspoon ras el hanout

1 tablespoon olive oil

2 garlic cloves, crushed

Salt and freshly ground black pepper

Grated zest of 1 lemon

5 scallions, finely sliced or shredded

2 tablespoons pomegranate molasses (optional)

1. Preheat the oven to 400°F (200°C).
2. Place the salmon, skin side down, on a large baking sheet lined with greased foil or parchment paper.
3. Mix the sumac with the ras el hanout, olive oil, garlic, and salt and pepper in a small bowl to make a paste. Rub evenly over the surface of the salmon to coat.
4. Bake for 15 minutes, or until the fish is cooked and will flake easily when tested with the tip of a knife.
5. Remove from the oven and sprinkle with the lemon zest, scallions, and pomegranate molasses, if using. Serve hot or cold.

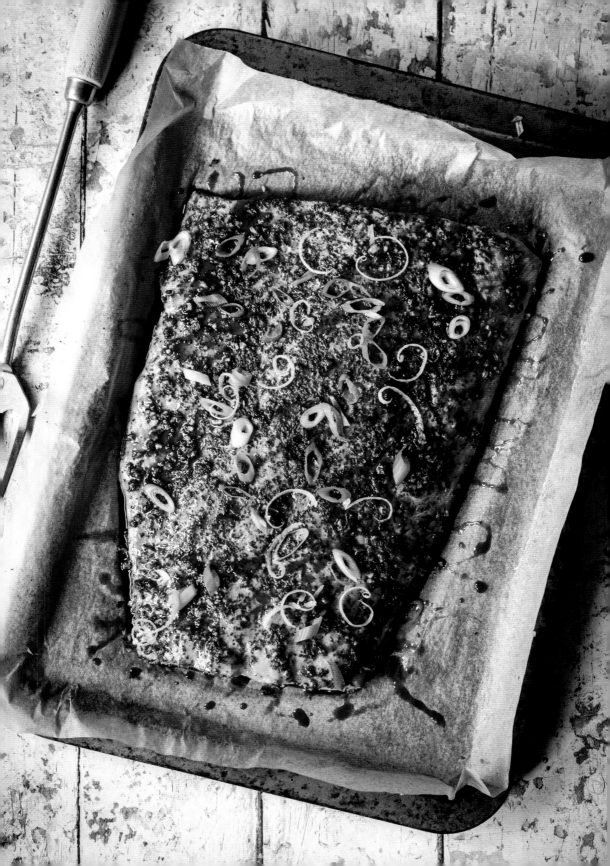

Gingered Ham

This flavorful ham is slow-cooked in the oven, resulting in meltingly tender meat with a sticky ginger glaze. It's a favorite at Christmastime but can be rolled out for any seasonal celebration. It will comfortably serve eight or more.

			SERVES **8**	
PER PORTION:	CALORIES **470**	PROTEIN **62.4 g**	CARBOHYDRATE **2.6 g**	FAT **23.4 g**

6½ pounds (3 kg) boneless ham

2½ cups (750 ml) sugar-free ginger beer

1 onion, quartered

Small piece ginger, peeled and sliced

10 black peppercorns

6 whole cloves

1 tablespoon grated peeled fresh ginger

3 tablespoons reduced-sugar ginger jam, jelly, or marmalade, or orange marmalade

Extra cloves, to decorate (optional)

1. Preheat the oven to 320°F (160°C). Place the ham in a deep roasting pan that will snugly hold it. Add all but ⅓ cup (75 ml) of the ginger beer to the ham along with the onion, sliced ginger, peppercorns, and cloves. Cover tightly with a double layer of foil and bake for 4½ hours, basting once or twice.

2. Uncover and pour away all but 1 tablespoon of the juices from the ham. Increase the oven temperature to 400°F (200°C).

3. To make the glaze, heat the remaining ginger beer with the grated ginger and ginger jam, until boiling. Reduce the heat and simmer for 5 minutes, until syrupy.

4. Meanwhile, cut away any skin from the ham, leaving just a thin layer of fat. Score the fat into a diamond pattern and brush over half the glaze. Decorate the cut surface with studded cloves, if desired. Return to the oven and roast, uncovered, for 10 minutes.

5. Brush again with the remaining glaze, and roast for a further 10 to 15 minutes, until golden. Serve hot or cold.

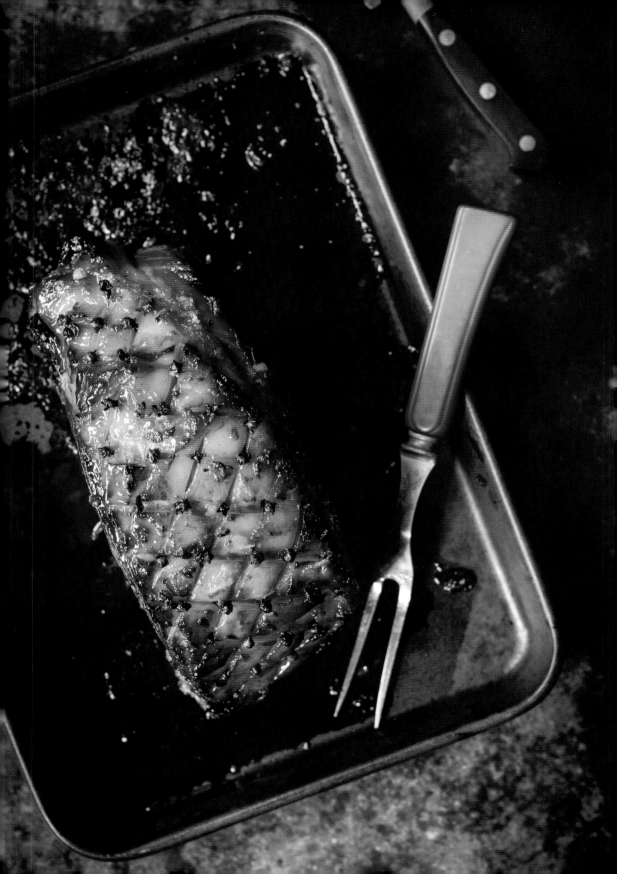

Bittersweet Winter Salad

WLS PORTION: ¼–½

This is a salad to serve in the autumn or winter months at a celebratory gathering (like Thanksgiving, Christmas, or New Year's Eve). Use tangerines or clementines; Belgian endive or radicchio; walnuts or pecans; and tarragon, mint, or cilantro, in any combination you like. It goes well with any deli meats, and is great on a buffet table.

	SERVES 4		V
PER PORTION:	CALORIES 270	PROTEIN 7.3 g	CARBOHYDRATE 11.6 g	FAT 20.5 g

1 small red onion, thinly sliced into rings

1 garlic clove, thinly sliced

Juice of 1 lemon

½ cup (50 g) walnut or pecan halves

3 heads Belgian endive or radicchio, leaves separated

6 to 8 clementines, tangerines, or satsumas, peeled and sliced

4 ounces (100 g) feta cheese, crumbled

2 tablespoons olive oil

Salt and freshly ground black pepper

1 to 2 tablespoons chopped fresh tarragon, mint, or cilantro

1. Place the red onion and garlic in a bowl with the lemon juice and set aside for 10 minutes.
2. Meanwhile, toast the walnuts or pecans in a dry frying pan for 2 to 3 minutes, until the skins have darkened and split. Crush lightly or roughly chop.
3. Arrange the endive or radicchio and fruit slices on a serving plate. Lift the onion and garlic from the lemon juice with a slotted spoon and scatter over the chicory and fruit slices with the cheese and nuts.
4. Whisk the oil into the lemon juice with salt and pepper to taste, and drizzle over the salad. Scatter over the herbs to serve.

Fluffy Easter Lemon Mousse

It's the sharp tang of lemon that makes this light-as-air mousse irresistible. It makes a great dessert recipe for Easter eating. You could add 3 tablespoons limoncello to the Quark for an especially indulgent dessert.

○ ● ● | SERVES **6**

PER PORTION:	CALORIES **111**	PROTEIN **12.2 g**	CARBOHYDRATE **4.7 g**	FAT **4.8 g**

2 unwaxed lemons

1 envelope unflavored gelatin

4 large eggs, separated

4 tablespoons granulated sweetener (or to taste)

8 ounces (250 g) fat-free quark, or low-fat soft cheese

Grated lemon zest, to decorate

1. Using a fine grater, grate the zest from the lemons into a bowl. Squeeze the juice from the lemons and set aside.
2. Place the gelatin in a small bowl, add the lemon juice, and allow to "sponge" or swell for 10 minutes.
3. Meanwhile, place the egg yolks, sweetener, and lemon zest in a bowl, and whisk until pale and light.
4. Set the bowl of gelatin in or over a pan of simmering water and leave until melted and clear. Alternatively, this can be done in the microwave by heating for 30 seconds. Let cool.
5. Beat 7 ounces (200 g) of the quark until smooth, then fold in the egg yolk mixture. Stir in the cooled dissolved gelatin.
6. Whisk the egg whites until stiff, then gently fold into the lemon mixture. Spoon into 1 large bowl or 6 small serving glasses, level the surface, and chill to set, about 3 hours.
7. Serve decorated with small spoonfuls of the remaining quark and a little grated lemon zest.

Meringue Wreath

Here's a show-stopping grand finale dessert for serving over the festive Thanksgiving, Christmas, or New Year's period. I've given three alternative ways of preparing—one as the usual sugar meringue (if you're not sugar-sensitive), the second as a sweetener-type meringue, and the third as an extra-speedy version using ready-made meringue nests. The first and third should be eaten with caution if you are very sugar-sensitive, but should be fine if only having a very small portion. The sweetener version (which most WLS patients can tolerate) makes a meringue that is very soft and marshmallow-like. You can decorate as flamboyantly as you like with fruit (frosted perhaps?), chocolate leaves, shards of edible gold leaf, and extravagant bows or curled citrus rind to add the final festive touch.

SUGAR VERSION/SWEETENER VERSION:	CALORIES 130/80	PROTEIN 7.4 g/8.5 g	CARBOHYDRATE 22 g/8.3 g	FAT 0.5 g/0.4 g

SERVES **8** — Ⓥ

6 large egg whites

1³/₄ cups (350 g) confectioners' sugar or ½ cup (100 g) granulated sweetener

2 teaspoons white wine vinegar

1 teaspoon vanilla extract

2 tablespoons dried cranberries

1 pound (450 g) quark or low-fat soft cheese, or fat-free Greek yogurt

Salted caramel or vanilla extract, to taste

Extra dried cranberries, holly leaves, orange zest, and a bow, to decorate (optional)

2 tablespoons sugar-free or low-sugar chocolate syrup, to drizzle (optional)

1. Preheat the oven to 250°F (120°C). Draw a 10-inch (25 cm) circle on a large sheet of parchment paper as a guide for the wreath circle, and place on a baking sheet.

2. Whisk the egg whites until they form stiff peaks, then whisk in the sugar or 5 tablespoons of the sweetener, 1 tablespoon at a time, whisking well between additions, until the mixture is thick, stiff, and glossy. Fold in the vinegar and vanilla extract with a metal spoon.

3. Spoon the meringue into ovals on the paper, using the circle as a guideline. Sprinkle with the dried cranberries.

4. Bake for 30 minutes. Reduce the heat to 225°F (110°C) and bake for an additional 1½ hours. Turn off the oven, open the door, and leave the meringue to cool completely.

5. To serve, beat the quark or yogurt with the remaining sweetener (or a little extra sugar, if desired) and salted caramel or vanilla extract to taste. Spoon this over the meringue in dollops and decorate with a few extra dried cranberries, holly leaves, orange zest, and a bow. Drizzle with the chocolate syrup just before serving, if desired.

SPEEDY VERSION: Use 8 ready-made meringue nests instead of the meringue mixture above, and sandwich or position together with a little of the quark mixture, using the remainder to fill the nests. Sprinkle with dried cranberries, then decorate and drizzle as above.

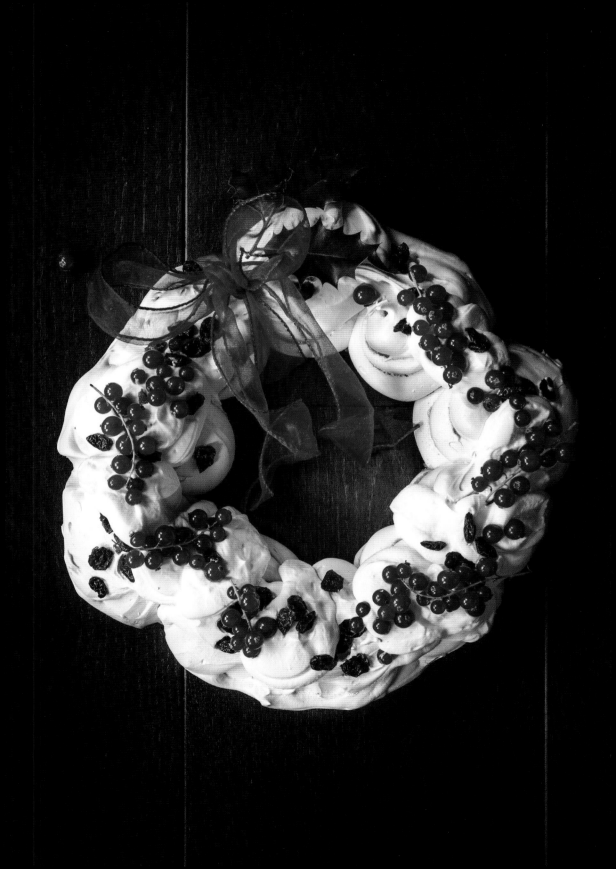

Crustless Pumpkin Pie

Come Thanksgiving, most WLS patients don't usually miss out on the turkey but often have to forego the sweet pies. This pumpkin one addresses that issue because you can enjoy it without a pastry crust. Remember to use pure canned pumpkin rather than a sweetened pie version for this recipe.

	SERVES 6	V

PER PORTION:	CALORIES 132	PROTEIN 8.2 g	CARBOHYDRATE 14.4 g	FAT 5.1 g

15-ounce (425 g) can pure pumpkin

½ cup (100 g) granulated sweetener

1 teaspoon ground cinnamon

½ teaspoon ground ginger

¼ teaspoon ground cloves

Pinch of salt

2 eggs

One 12-ounce (300 g) can evaporated skim milk

Sugar-free, low-fat whipped topping, to serve (optional)

1. Preheat the oven to 300°F (150°C).
2. Mix the pumpkin with the sweetener, cinnamon, ginger, cloves, and salt. Beat in the eggs, one at a time, until well-blended. Stir in the evaporated milk and mix well.
3. Pour into a deep 9-inch (23 cm) deep-dish pie plate and bake for 30 to 35 minutes, until set but still a little wobbly in the center.
4. Remove from the oven and allow to cool to room temperature. Serve warm, or cool and then chill. Cut into wedges to serve, topped with a little sugar-free, low-fat whipped topping, if desired.

TIP: The uncooked pumpkin mixture can be poured into a premade pastry or graham cracker cookie crust and then baked, if preferred. Bake in a preheated 350°F (180°C) oven for 30 to 35 minutes.

Christmas Punch

WLS
PORTION:
½–1

I have often been asked to come up with a fruity punch idea that is suitable for bariatrics to imbibe during the festivities. Here is one of my favorite nonalcoholic ones made with red tea, pomegranate juice, and spices. If you wish to reduce the sugar content per serving, simply add more water or diet ginger ale to the punch, and stir well to release as many bubbles as you possibly can. For those who wish, alcohol of your choice can be added.

● ● ●		SERVES **4**		**V**
PER PORTION (with regular/light juice):	CALORIES **40/9**	PROTEIN **0.1 g/0.1 g**	CARBOHYDRATE **9.6 g/1.6 g**	FAT **0 g/0 g**

2 rooibos tea bags

1 teaspoon granulated sweetener

6 whole cloves

1 cinnamon stick

1¼ cups (300 ml) regular pomegranate juice or light pomegranate and blueberry juice

Sliced plums and lemon wedges, to decorate (optional)

1. Put the tea bags, sweetener, cloves, and cinnamon stick into a large heatproof jug and pour over 2½ cups (600 ml) boiling water. Let stand for 5 minutes, then strain into a serving jug.
2. Add the pomegranate juice and stir well to mix.
3. Serve in glasses decorated with plum slices and lemon wedges, if desired.

Eggnog for Bariatrics

Is it even possible to make an eggnog that is bariatric-friendly? One that isn't overloaded with sugar, fat, and alcohol? Well, yes, it's possible to make the classic one a tad more healthy, but it won't be really low in fat nor totally sugar-free. But if eggnog is on your must-have list at holiday time, this is a better option. Perhaps just stick with one glass (a dainty small one at that)? The alcohol, of course, is optional.

● ● ●	SERVES 6			V
PER PORTION (using sugar, but not rum):	CALORIES 99	PROTEIN 6.9 g	CARBOHYDRATE 10.6 g	FAT 3.4 g

3 eggs, separated
2 tablespoons sugar or granulated sweetener
½ teaspoon vanilla extract
3 cups (700 ml) low-fat milk
¼ cup plus 2 tablespoons (90 ml) rum (optional)
Grated nutmeg, to dust

1. Beat the egg yolks with the sugar or sweetener. Stir in the vanilla, milk, and rum, if using.
2. Beat the egg whites until stiff but moist peaks form, and fold into the egg yolk mixture.
3. Pour into small glasses and sprinkle the tops with grated nutmeg.

Acknowledgments

As with all books, there are more people involved in the conception and production of the publication than the author's name on the jacket. This is most definitely true of this book. Since its aim has been to impart all the knowledge I have learned, and wise words I have been given over the years since my surgery, it has a vast list of contributors who have added to that experience.

Many of these are professional friends and colleagues in the health, obesity, and food world; my sponsors on the website and Bariatric Cookery Newsletter, without whom it wouldn't be possible to continue to provide free and unbiased information; my website designers, "protectors," and "upgraders;" professional and amateur cooks who help with my tweaking of recipes; charity and campaigning groups with obesity care at their core; press and PR personnel who help and support with sourcing images and information; support group admins and their lively members who keep it real; my guest website contributors who specialize in subjects that I can only scratch the surface of, and allow me to bring to you the wealth of their experience and advice; other "bariatric experts" who realize we're a poorly funded and supported community, and so give their time and some features without fear of competitiveness (even though we compete to a certain extent in the same arena, we recognize that we're all in this together); and the new friends I have made along the way through WLS who now are life-long ones. My surgeon, Shaw Somers is still my "God" and probably always will be.

You will find a list of these below, and I only wish I could name every WLS patient who has been supportive, made me think hard, and shored things up when the going got tough (because even the adviser needs a helping hand occasionally). I think you know who you all are, and I salute you!

Some of the information in this book has also featured on my website, bariatriccookery.com, and the free newsletter—some of which has been written by guest contributors or other organizations, and for which I am eternally grateful to be able to share. Check out their websites for more detailed information. Bariatrics is still a new science and much is being added to it in terms of research on a daily basis. Many WLS patients often become "experts by experience" and can be proactive with their research, too—don't ever close your mind or think "job done."

I am also grateful to my UK publishers Grub Street, whom I have known for many years. I thank them for having the belief in a book on a controversial subject like weight loss surgery, and for being open-minded and forward-thinking.

Thanks also to my US editor, Olivia Peluso, and everyone else at The Experiment for believing in this book and spreading the message to an American audience. Of course, this is always a team effort, so many thanks, too, to the publisher, Matthew Lore; art director, Beth Bugler; designer, Jack Dunnington; and managing editor, Zach Pace.

Huge thanks must also go to photographer Regula Ysewijn and food stylist Kathy Kordalis, who have made each and every recipe look effortlessly beautiful. I am such a fussy and hard to please food stylist myself, and I love each and every one of them, which speaks volumes!

Last but not least I must thank my family—my husband, Peter, who really is the backbone to this bariatric set-up, with his unstinting support, and taking on duties that involve admin, accounting, ordering, shipping products, blog picture-taking . . . and, for light relief, recipe sampling. Thank you to my daughter, Lucinda, son, Charlie, and son-in-law, Stephen, for professional PR and IT help (lessening stress appreciably in the face of adversity). They all put up with a lot when this book was "cooking."

Resources

Nathan Lewis, Toni Jenkins (specialist bariatric consultant), and Nichola Ludlam-Raine (dietician) at Ramsay Healthcare
ramsayhealth.co.uk

Kerry Cooper at Baricol Vitamins
baricol.com

Shaw Somers, Guy Slater, and Chris Pring (surgeons) and Sue Smith at Streamline Surgical
streamline-surgical.com

Dr Connie Stapleton (psychologist)
conniestapletonphd.com

Alex Brechner at BariatricPal
BariatricPal.com

Lisa Kaouk and Monica Bashaw (dieticians) at Bariatric Surgery Nutrition
bariatricsurgerynutrition.com

James Brooks at Brooks Creative
brookscreative.co

Steph Wagner at Food Coach Me
foodcoach.me

Scott Lonnee (bariatric dietitian) at St George's Hospital, Tooting, London

Ken Clare, Bianca Scollen, Angela Brown plus all other team members of WLSinfo.org Charity
wlsinfo.org.uk

Lesley McCormack, Lynne Potter, and all the other team members at HOOP (Helping Overcome Obesity Problems) Charity
hoop.uk.org.uk

Dr Sally Norton (surgeon) at Vavista
vavistalife.com

Owen Haskins at Bariatric News
bariatricnews.net

Professor Paul Gately at Leeds Beckett University and MoreLife
leedsbeckett.ac.uk

The Obesity Action Coalition (OAC)
obesityaction.org

American Society For Metabolic and Bariatric Surgery
asmbs.org

Shape Up America
shapeup.org

Tam Fry at the National Obesity Forum
nationalobesityforum.org.uk

Dan Abeling at Obesity Coverage
obesitycoverage.com

Cheryl Anne Borne at My Bariatric Life
mybariatriclife.org

Kristen Willard (dietician) at Bariatric Meal Prep
bariatricmealprep.com

Neil Floch (surgeon) and Burton Zaretsky at Fairfield County Bariatrics
endtheweight.com

Subject Index

Recipe Index

NOTE: Page numbers in *italics* indicate a photograph.

About the Author

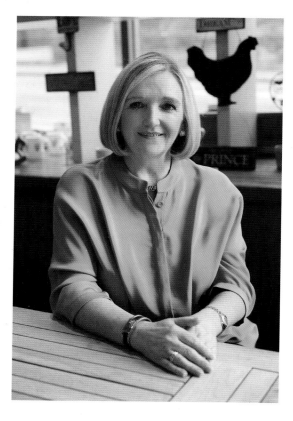

CAROL BOWEN BALL is a professional bariatric cook, having undergone weight loss surgery ten years ago. She helps those who have had (or are considering) weight loss surgery to achieve long-lasting success with flavorful recipes and expert lifestyle advice. She has written over ninety cookbooks on a variety of subjects, from barbecue to range-style cooking. She lives in Camberley, England.

bariatriccookery.com